With Liberty and Coverage for All

Who shall live, who shall die and how to survive under Obamacare

Thomas A. Sharon, R.N., M.P.H.

Sharon Books

Copyright © 2012 Thomas A. Sharon, R.N., M.P.H.

Sharon Books

Bay Harbor Islands, Florida

305-705-7869

All rights reserved.

ISBN-10: 1479305154

ISBN-13: 978-1479305155

Dedication

To:

My dear wife Naomi

My beloved children:

Kimberly

Dana

Ria

Ramon

Monica

Isadora

My mother, Frances Ginsberg of blessed memory

Acknowledgements

With gratitude to the leaders of the Institute of Medicine for their truthful disclosure of the dismal state of health care in the United States

With gratitude to the anonymous physicians and scientists in the F.D.A. who blew the whistle on the widespread corruption and abuse of power in the agency, for their integrity, patriotism and courage.

Table of Contents

Introduction..6

1 The Insidious Plan—Targeting Seniors........................14

2 Medical Mistakes..34

3 The Never Ending Story of Never Events.....................62

4 Hospital Mistakes: the Root Causes and the Cures.............84

5 The Socialist Agenda and the AMA Capitulation.............102

6 Medical Politics and Political Medicine...........................123

7 Healthcare Reform: First do no Harm............................143

8 Reinventing the Reinvented Wheel................................161

9 From Lip to Law..185

10 The Political Pretext..206

11 The Death Panel Shell Game......................................230

12 Health Care "Reform" in 2010....................................248

13 FDA = Fraud, Deception and Abuse...........................263

14 The Medicinal Mayhem...292

15 PPACA – the Roadmap to Chaos...............................314

16 The New National Priorities for Health Care Reform.........338

17 The Baby Boomers' Survival Guide..............................370

Introduction

The current state of health care is in shambles with doctors and nurses accidentally killing more patients than most of the diseases they are treating. The new law has failed to protect the public with patient safety standards, and will soon head us toward a condition of total financial collapse and chaos with thousands of hospitals and clinics closed down and millions of people dying of treatable diseases.

Therefore, to avert this inevitable disaster this book proposes both political and personal solutions such as legislating patient safety standards and staying off the "who shall die" lists with interventions for prevention. Once the Government moves us into a single payer system it will have only one choice to save itself from disintegration; to keep spiraling health care costs under control by preventing the old and disabled from receiving expensive life-saving hospital care. Thus the health care industry, which already has an oversight system in place for pre-authorization of high-priced medical services, supplies, equipment and drugs, will provide only to government-approved recipients after the panels of bureaucrats make their decision on who shall live and who shall die.

There is no question that we have been lied to and victimized in what is probably the greatest scam in history. But it didn't just start with Obama's election and the passing of the Patient Protection and Affordable Care Act of 2010; it started decades ago with the advent of the health maintenance organization that forever changed the face of medical practice and health care delivery in the United States.

The Third Biggest Lie

We used to say the two biggest lies are "The check is in the mail" and "It won't hurt a bit." Now, there is a third biggest lie, which is, "We have the best health care system in the world," as Bill Clinton, George Bush and Barak Obama have uttered repeatedly during their respective terms. On the other hand, all of the standard measures of health care quality points to ours as being "the best substandard price-gouging health care system in the world". One such measure is a comparison of cost and longevity[1]. For example, Americans live an average of 77 years at a cost of $4,800 per person per year, while Spain, Canada and Japan respectively have life span-to-cost ratios of 79 years at $1,100, 81.5 years at $2,100, and 81 years at $2,000.

Another measure is the infant death rate per one thousand live births and the U.S. has a rate comparable to third world countries at 6.9 compared to 5.3 in Denmark, 4.6 in France, 3.4 in Sweden and 3.2 in Japan. Additionally, the World Health Organization ranks the United States as 37th in the world, which puts us just behind Costa Rica.

Therefore, we can see that the people of other countries get better outcomes for much less cost, suggesting that we Americans are paying more for inferior quality products and services. Although President Obama and other politicians acknowledge that health care is too expensive, they have been downplaying the fact that organized medicine in the United States has been giving the public a royal hosing for decades.

---

[1] http://www.infoplease.com/ipa/A0934556.html

Introduction

What's Really Wrong with Health Care

Some of the problems with U.S. health care delivery as many other experts have also pointed out are as follows:

1. Hospitals, nursing homes and clinics are unsafe with medical and nursing negligence being the fifth largest cause of death in the United States.
2. Lack of access with 76 million uninsured (adding illegal aliens) and 106 million underinsured;
3. Out of control costs with health care being 16% of gross domestic product (GDP) at $1 trillion which is a 250% increase over the last 25 years;
4. Price gouging, with hospitals and doctors charging uninsured patients 1000% more than they accept from third party payers;
5. HMO premium price gouging with high deductibles charging 300% more for individuals who purchase directly rather than through a group;
6. Health care corporations are guilty of bilking billions of dollars from tax payers with fraudulent billing practices;
7. Doctors perform unnecessary surgery with bogus diagnoses;
8. H.M.O. members have to call for approval before going to emergency rooms with call centers outsourced to non-professional personnel in India and other countries;
9. Administrative cost of DRG's and CPT codes is $375 billion per year – 25% of total health care expenditures;
10. Pharmaceutical companies obtain FDA approval for toxic drugs by paying large research grants to medical research facilities to achieve favorable results;
11. Pharmaceutical companies pay bribes to physicians to

prescribe their over-priced toxic drugs with tens of thousands falling prey to side effects causing injury and death.

This short list of scams and rackets is really the largest, most harmful and costly criminal conspiracy in history. The perpetrators include HMO's, pharmaceutical companies, hospital and physician groups and politicians. Additionally, with the political corruption achieved through expensive lobbying to defeat all attempts to impose regulatory standards, we can see why we pay such exorbitant prices for such shabby health care.

How we got into this Mess

To explain further, medical care has always been a business whereby the seller decides what the consumer will purchase and how much. Couple that control with fear of death, and the buyer will pay any price for care on any terms. Hence there is complete command and control and the public will accept any propaganda that will calm their fears of putting their lives in the hands of incompetent corporate executives who are interested only in maximizing profits. Moreover, the people of our generation and the previous one grew up trusting our doctors and listening for the most part, to what they recommended. Then medicine evolved moving from cottage industry to commercial empires.

However, to our disadvantage, we still had this mindset of "doctor knows best" for decades while the entire paradigm of ethics changed to acceptance of greedy commercialism with corporate executives capturing financial control of health care operations and finding ways to deny coverage for expensive services and equipment rentals with the pre-approval requirement fraud. Once a well-meaning physician prescribes a treatment, a non-professional decides whether it is medically necessary. Physicians, who became financially dependent upon their corporate "bosses", would have to capitulate. Then Congress stepped in and gave legislative immunity to HMO's from lawsuits for wrongful death and damages caused by withholding approval for life-sustaining treatment[2], thus leaving the doctors and hospitals holding the proverbial bag with malpractice lawsuits. The whole scenario was like putting a hungry shark in a pond to take care of the fish. The shark, knowing that if he swallows everyone in one gulp he won't last long, says to each of his group members, "There is something wrong with the way your tail is functioning so I'm going to have to bite part of it off for your own good," and the tasty fish replies, "You're the doctor."

The False Solutions

Moreover, there have been some suggested health care reform models coming from various think tanks such as "public good", which is government provided or contracted care, versus the "public utility model", being privately owned health care with quality standards and pricing controlled by a government agency like public utilities. Although we have seen a lot of pundits and politicians arguing the pros and cons for both and, notwithstanding that we have a new health reform law taking

---

[2] The U.S. congress granted Immunity from liability in malpractice lawsuits to managed care companies and HMO's providing health care plans purchased through employers through the passing of the federal Employee Retirement Income Savings Act of 1974 (ERISA). Internet resource:
http://www.ncbi.nlm.nih.gov/pmc/articles/PMC2608383/pdf/jnma00365-0019.pdf)

effect, we are still lacking a viable solution.

On the other hand, to have a workable infrastructure, we will need to abandon those policies that have ended in disaster, such as using financial incentives to control physician behavior, defining health care as providing diagnostics, drugs and surgery and autocratic corporate control of treatment plans. Furthermore, we have to stop believing in this myth called "freedom of choice" as if there was any free choice in health care to begin with. This term has become a way to placate us into accepting a crappy plan charging us more for less by saying, "We have preserved your freedom to choose." So what if I don't like the pond that I'm swimming in? I can look for another one with a different shark.

The Socialist Agenda

Yet, there is now another fiddle that came from Washington, D.C. called "The Patient Protection Affordable Care Act of 2010." The president and his political hacks in Congress say they have revolutionized the health care industry by making it cheaper, better, more accessible and safer. The problem is that this administration and its pork barrel Congress has no clue as to what preventable errors cause the unnecessary killing of 200,000 people annually in hospitals across the country, and even if they wanted to stop the carnage they wouldn't be able to figure out how.

The Mirage

The new Patient Protection and Affordable Care Act of 2010 is a sham. It looks like there is going to be more access to health care plans at lower cost, but it's a mirage. First of all, the table of contents in the 974-page law document is all screwed up so it will take all day to find any particular section. There are also

Introduction

a myriad of confusing amendments and add-ons that have nothing to do with the so-called health insurance changes so there is a huge hurdle in trying to understand this new statute. However, we do know that the law will require everyone to purchase a private health plan and the insurance companies won't be allowed to turn anyone down for any reason. The mandate for healthy people to buy insurance is a joke. Even if the Feds can enforce a $750 fine it would be cheaper than paying premiums. Only those who need health care will sign up. Obviously the private carriers, who are now price gouging the public to get what they can while they can get it, will disappear, leaving the Government in control of all health services as the single payer.

Meanwhile, the new law deliberately leaves about 30 million people still uninsured, which gives the Government an excuse to add a "public option" to the mix, which will be a precursor to the planned single payer system.

Finally, as we listen to the political rhetoric about the current state of health care and how to improve it, we get a sense that it's not so bad and we can make it better. On the contrary, when we go to a hospital as a patient or to visit and we see that people have to wait thirty minutes for a bed pan to avoid soiling themselves, we wake up to a different reality in the world of chaos. Therefore, as we examine the new health care reform scheme, we can quickly ascertain that our elected officials have opted to put more fish in the ponds and tell the sharks to take smaller bites.

Therefore, this book is about exposing the greatest political scam and rip-off conspiracy that the world has ever seen and how we might navigate through the world of impending chaos. We begin by understanding the political agenda and the plan. Then we shall move to unravel the mysteries of the new law to foresee the new bureaucratic structure that will decide who shall live and who shall die. We all need to know where each of us is likely to land in those identifying categories that will determine whether we will be granted access to expensive medical treatment or condemned to hospice; the new death row of the disenfranchised and the gateway to euthanasia.

1. The Insidious Plan—Targeting Seniors

Life and Death

Health care is a matter of life or death and to stay alive, we all have to purchase expensive professional services and products at various times and most of us can't afford it. Therefore, in order to ensure that we can get health care when we need it, we have to pay for it when we don't need it. Hence, we have health plans. It was an idea that worked in principle with an entire population paying into a pool; the healthy would pay for the sick and the management company would reap the profits. However, as the cost of health care continued to spiral so did the cost of the health plan premiums leaving more and more people struggling to maintain some level of coverage, which has been eroding with widening gaps in the way of larger and larger deductibles, with about 30% of every health care dollar being spent on administration and bottom line.

Accordingly, the age-old debate in the United States is whether or not every citizen and legal resident is entitled to all that one's condition requires to stay alive regardless of the cost. The moral standard is clear; life is sacred and almost everyone wants to live. Who wouldn't pay anything to keep oneself or a loved one alive and relieve the suffering? On the other hand, there is the pragmatic standard that the good of the many outweighs the good of the few, which is also a sound moral principle from the viewpoint of leadership. That's why we expect our presidents to send our young men and women into harm's way whenever there is a foreign or domestic threat to our national sovereignty.

Moreover, using the desperate need for life-saving treatment and invoking the idea of choosing a few to die so that many could live, government officials can utilize the health care system as an effective tool for command and control. The idea of a health care system that by design systematically causes the deaths of hundreds of thousands of people per year and injuring three times that many is so off the scale terrifying that the public couldn't accept it as truth even when the government blew the whistle on itself. The leaders of IOM broadcast to the world in a published book with a huge fanfare of publicity that our health care system was methodically killing 100,000 annually because of its design and management and did nothing in response but spend more than a billion dollars conducting useless studies.

In short, the policy of three administrations over eleven years was to study the problem and watch two million people die, with a majority of them being senior citizens. The fact that there has been no change in this degenerate policy through several shifts of power bouncing like a ping pong ball between the Democrats and Republicans suggests an even more insidious aspect to this plot; a shadow government with continuous command and control over executive policy.

The Start

Through the last sixty-five years since the end of World War II, our society developed a three-tier health care system; public coverage, private coverage and no coverage. Universal single payer found its way into the fold, but only for certain segments of the population such as veterans, people over the age of sixty-five, folks with disabilities and welfare recipients. By 1965, we had Medicare, Medicaid, the Veterans' Administration and the U.S. Public Health Service each in its own right becoming a huge bureaucracy with an army of paid personnel to provide health care services and administrative oversight. Additionally, over the last three decades, although each of those subsystems suffered budget cuts and austerity measures in the face of spiraling prices, the system remained static with a growing deterioration in quality of care, forcing health care personnel to make do with shortages of manpower, supplies and equipment.

The Progression

Additionally, while the government was trying desperately to hold down the price gouging, changing institutional reimbursement from fee-for-service to "prospective payment"[3], the private sector began instituting its innovative methods by selling health plans. They would contract with doctors and hospitals for cheaper prices and offer to provide all necessary health care as long as the member of the plan used preferred providers in the network. Unfortunately this plan backfired because prices continued to grow at ten times the broader inflation rate and the doctors controlled consumer demand. The only logical response was to take over total control of the doctors, so the large corporate insurance giants bought up the hospitals and medical practices. Those that wanted to remain self-

---

[3] https://www.cms.gov/ProspMedicareFeeSvcPmtGen/ "A Prospective Payment System (PPS) is a method of reimbursement in which Medicare payment is made based on a predetermined, fixed amount. The payment amount for a particular service is derived based on the classification system of that service (for example, diagnosis-related groups for inpatient hospital services). CMS uses separate PPSs for reimbursement to acute inpatient hospitals, home health agencies, hospice, hospital outpatient, inpatient psychiatric facilities, inpatient rehabilitation facilities, long-term care hospitals, and skilled nursing facilities."

employed signed provider agreements in order not to be left out of the patient referral machines. Hence, the Insurance companies became the health care providers and they quickly set up the pre-approval process whereby they could make decisions on whether they would pay for any type of treatment. In order to systematize the bases for denials, computer wonks designed software that would make algorithmic medical necessity decisions on who shall live and who shall die.

The Start of Rationing

Then health care kept getting more and more expensive with the development of new technology like magnetic resonance imaging (MRI), computerized tomography (CAT) scans, and designer drugs. Information technology also came into the act with digitized records that included all diagnostic information including X-ray images. Diagnostic blood and microbiology tests also jumped into the fast lane with hi-tech computer-driven processes adding to the ever growing costs. And, we now have computer driven DNA profiling technology at the cutting edge to determine the predictability of favorable responses to treatment.

The new price tags for the technological explosion are going to lead to financial implosion because it's more than we can afford. It's sucking us dry and the simple truth is that even if there is an available treatment that can save everyone who has a particular life-threatening condition, there just isn't enough money to pay for everyone who needs it.

The costs of Medicare doubled every four years between 1966 and 1980. According to the 2004 "Green Book" of the House Ways and Means Committee, Medicare expenditures from the American government were $256.8 billion in fiscal year 2002 while paid in premiums totaled $230.9 billion leaving an annual deficit of $25.9 billion.[4] The present value of unfunded obligations under all parts of Medicare during fiscal-year 2009 is approximately $36 trillion, which is more than three times the annual output of the entire U.S. economy[5].

Hence, the Medicare debt, which will increase at least tenfold by the time all the baby boomers become eligible in the next ten years, is going to collapse the U.S. economy and there is nothing that the government can do about it short of changing the moral paradigm to deny medical treatment for treatable diseases for the elderly and mentally disabled. The new questions of eligibility will be, "What is a life worth?" and "Is this life worth saving?"

Therefore, the preapproval process will inevitably evolve into creating death lists for those whose profiles don't make the grade for the cost/benefit ratio. Expensive medicines and treatments will be reserved for those for whom the probability bean counter machines (cost-to-benefit ratio calculator software) assign the best possible outcomes to those who are most likely to return to tax-paying productivity. DNA profiling will undoubtedly play a significant role.

The Bean-Counter Illustration

To illustrate, my late mother lived for seven more years after she fractured her hip at age 91. The cost of her health care was about $350,000, without which she would not have lived

---

[4]

http://en.wikipedia.org/wiki/Medicare_(United_States)#Costs_and_funding_challenges

[5] The 2009 Annual Report of the Board of Trustees of the Federal Old-Age and Survivors Insurance and Federal Disability Insurance Trust Funds.

beyond her hip fracture. It is painfully obvious that in the new order of health care that awaits us all, some government bean-counter is going to decide that $350,000 is not worth keeping a 91-year-old woman alive for 7 more years. It won't matter that a mother and son can benefit from seven more years of quality time because it doesn't produce revenue.

Moreover, the same bean-counters are going to come to the conclusion that it's not worth one million dollars per person to keep a 65-year-old man or woman alive for the next twenty years. Where will it stop? Will there be a government mandate to yank the plug on life-support if it has to last for more than three days? Add all of the bean-counter scenarios to the current wrongful death rates in health facilities and we can see that the health care centers of America are fast becoming killing fields.

The Baby Boomer Bubble is About to Burst

The first question in understanding any conspiracy is "Why?" Why would the government policy wonks decide to do nothing about the unsafe practices and methodologies in American health care facilities? Admittedly, it sounds crazy but the medical mishaps and hospital mistakes are increasing and causing more and more fatalities, with seniors over age 65 being more vulnerable and the do-nothing policy continues with more money squandered on "studying the problem." Thus the question stands; "Why?" In this case, the logical answer is the post-World War II baby-boom.

When we look at the age statistics from the Census Bureau, we can easily see that from 1998 to 2008, the U.S. population aged 65 and over increased by 15 percent, while the population aged 45 to 64 increased by 37 percent. The proportion of persons aged 65 and over is expected to increase in the future as the baby boomers, currently in the 45–64 age bracket, enter their elder years. In ten years, the baby boomer generation will consume about 70 percent of all prescription medications and the overall healthcare expenditures will at least double with most of it being spent on the thirty percent of the population that is over 65 years of age.

The people who control Medicare payment policy at the Centers for Medicare and Medicaid Services (CMS) have tried everything to keep the cost of senior health care from bankrupting this country. They have cut fees, caused hospitals to take flat rate reimbursement making it more profitable to discharge patients quicker and sicker, and slashed reimbursement to nursing homes and home care agencies causing massive numbers of facility closings leaving enormous shortages of beds and personnel. The result was a sharp increase in deaths related to neglect of disabled seniors; bedsores, choking, trauma from falling out of bed, abuse, dehydration and starvation.

Now, they refuse to pay for the additional hospital care needed to treat those complications and the scariest part of this revelation is that CMS has failed to contain the spiraling costs because the population of baby boomers keeps on getting older. The next step is unthinkable, but there is only one option left and Congress has taken it: cost-to-benefit ratio. The benefit consideration will have less to do with the chance of patient recovery and will rely more heavily on the individual's productivity index, based on age, earnings potential and the need for child-care services. The rest of us will get a free pass to go directly to hospice where they will make us "comfortable."

The Casualties: Two Million Dead and Still Counting

In 1999 the Institute of Medicine, a federal government agency, issued a lengthy report of medical mistakes called "To Err is Human." They stated that that there were supposedly 44,000 to 98,000 deaths annually due to medical errors.[6] Since Most hospitals and doctors who made fatal errors, kept their misadventures secret, the numbers, as scandalous as they sounded, were grossly understated. Moreover, the identification of the common medical mistakes barely scratched the surface, but was revealing some horrifying facts. The IOM officials stated, "The Quality of Health Care in America Committee of the Institute of Medicine (IOM) concluded that it is not acceptable for patients to be harmed by the health care system that is supposed to offer healing and comfort—a system that promises, "First, do no harm." Helping to remedy this problem was the goal of *To Err is Human: Building a Safer Health System*, the IOM Committee's first report."

The authors at IOM stated that faulty systems, processes, and conditions that lead people to make mistakes or fail to prevent them were the more common causes of errors. The "less common causes" were the recklessness of individual health care workers. In short, the United States Government reported in 1999 that nearly 100,000 people were being killed each year in the health care facilities throughout the United States due to dangerous life-threatening conditions and President Bill Clinton and the United States Congress did nothing to stop the carnage.

During mid-2004, Dr. Lucian Leape, co-author of To Err is Human, had stated publicly that there had been no significant improvement in patient safety in the five years since the IOM

---

[6] To Err Is Human: Building a Safer Health System; National Academies Press; 1st edition (April 15, 2000)

report was made public. This meant that another 500,000 Americans had lost their lives in a health care system that the Government had declared unsafe, and still no action was being contemplated. The bewildering aspect of this was that there was no press coverage.

In July, 2004, Healthgrades, Inc., a private company that evaluates the quality of hospitals and physician practices issued a report of the results of another government study conducted by the Agency for Healthcare Research and Quality (AHRQ) that showed an alarming number of deaths per year due to hospital mistakes alone that was much greater that the number published by the IOM in 1999. The government was not forthcoming with this information and if not for Healthgrades personnel, this information would have remain buried unpublished in the government archives. By this time, George Bush was the Republican president and the do nothing policy remained unchanged.

The AHRQ study of the Medicare population's health care experience between 2000 and 2002 revealed that a total of 1.14 million life-threatening mistakes occurred in approximately 37 million hospitalizations. These incidents resulted in 265,000 deaths just among the Medicare population alone. Therefore, the over-all population estimate of accidental killings was about 200,000 per year. The Healthgrades reports for subsequent years showed that we have been losing 200,000 Americans every year for ten years since the news of hospital mistakes broke loose in 1999. Our health care system, that politicians have been touting as the best in the world has killed more than 2 million people since 9/11/2001. That's more casualties than the Vietnam and the two Iraqi wars combined. Health Care itself is the fifth leading cause of death in the United States.

The risk of death by hospitalization today is one in five hundred and increasing. The members of Congress and the President know it and continue to do nothing because most of the victims are seniors. They all knew it eleven years ago when it became part of the public consciousness. The bipartisan policy decision is to continue to let people die from mistakes, equipment failures, shortages and deliberate neglect. The obvious reason is to reduce the population of baby boomers to a more financially manageable level.

The Government's Response: Study the Problem and Watch People Die

Talk about reinventing the wheel! The new health care reform legislation from Congress is supposed to establish some sort of bureaucracy that will attend to improve the quality of health care in America. I feel like I'm going insane because this department has already existed for at least twenty years; it's the Agency for Health Care Research and Quality, which is a division of the Department for Health and Human Services. Of course, since hospital care is the fifth leading cause of death in the United States, a fact that came to light ten years ago in an explosive media scandal, one has to wonder, "How much money has the Agency for Health Care Research and Quality spent on improving health care in the last ten years and why do we still end up with hundreds of thousands of health care victims every year? Based on this past performance, another big question that we have to ask is, "Why in the world would any sane person think that the government can reform health care, health insurance or anything else when its top elected and appointed officials are all scalawags, liars and thieves?

So, let's take a closer look at the Agency for Health Care

Research and Quality (AHRQ) to see what it's been up to lately. First we need to examine its mission statement:

"The Agency for Healthcare Research and Quality (AHRQ) sponsors research to improve the quality of health care in America. As part of the Department of Health and Human Services, AHRQ is tasked with elevating health care quality, reducing medical-related costs and expanding healthcare access for more Americans. Almost 80% of AHRQ's budget is awarded as grants and contracts to researchers at universities and other research institutions across the country. Early in its history, the agency became heavily involved in a controversial healthcare reform plan that almost led to AHRQ being eliminated. Since then, the agency has maintained a low profile, low on controversy."

So now we can clearly see that the AHRQ was nothing more than a conduit for funneling political graft to the tune of about $1 billion to fund phony research projects over the last ten years, while 2 million people lost their lives unnecessarily with 6 million more suffering catastrophic injuries. Meanwhile, in order to protect this money funneling scam, the present and past administrations told the AHRQ to refrain from rocking the boat.

The following is a list of the top ten of the 619 recipients from 2000 to 2008, who were supposed to find ways to improve the quality of health care[7]:

Westat, Inc.	$363,082,579
Social & Scientific Systems	$53,602,531
Research Triangle Institute	$43,532,123

---

[7]

http://www.allgov.com/Agency/Agency_for_Healthcare_Research_and_Quality

Emergency Care Research Institute	$31,423,379
National Opinion Research Center	$26,685,066
Thomson Company Inc.	$24,680,365
Oregon Health & Science University	$24,608,949
Booz Allen Hamilton Inc.	$24,231,318
Hopkins Johns University	$23,497,500
Rand Corporation	$16,442,390

As of this writing, I have no clue as to what those 619 private and public entities did with $1 billion of federal research grants for improving health care quality because there are now more unnecessary deaths and injuries than ever before. The saddest part of this commentary is that under the 2010 Patient Protection and Affordable Care Act, congress is slated to spend even more money to study the quality and access issues at an accelerated rate. Therefore we can only conclude that based on past performance any further government intervention will cause us to continue to pay more for less at a faster rate. The only way for the Obama administration to reverse this trend is to deny expensive treatment to most seniors. Death by denial of services will be an option to save money.

To continue, the AHRQ recently published the results of one of the studies that it funded. The report states that the number of hospital patient deaths in 2007 was 765,651. Twelve percent of those who died were in the hospital for elective procedures, fifteen percent died of hospital acquired blood infection, and a substantial number choked to death. The total amount of unnecessary deaths was thirty percent. The report also concluded that hospital bills are three times more costly for patients who expire than for patients who leave the hospital alive. Therefore, since the AHRQ reports that dying patients cost an average of $27,000 compared to $9,000 for live ones, if the hospitals will stop killing their patients, the system will save about 3.6 billion dollars per year.

On the other hand, since a patient who dies brings in three times more revenue to a hospital that a patient who survives, one begins to wonder if the overall financial incentive lends itself to repetitive incidences of unexpected protracted illness followed by premature death.

Furthermore, since improved patient safety would reduce government expenditures for hospital care by 3.6 billion dollars per year, one has to wonder why AHRQ found it necessary to maintain a low profile for the agency to survive. Why would three different administrations continuously choose to do nothing and tell the people at AHRQ personnel to keep their mouths shut?

The Agency for Healthcare Research and Quality (AHRQ) has stated on their website, "Medical errors are one of the Nation's leading causes of death and injury."
Here is how they define medical error:

"Medical errors happen when something that was planned as a part of medical care doesn't work out, or when the wrong plan was used in the first place. Medical errors can occur anywhere in the health care system:
- Hospitals.
- Clinics.
- Outpatient Surgery Centers.
- Doctors' Offices.
- Nursing Homes.
- Pharmacies.
- Patients' Homes.

Errors can involve:
- Medicines.

- Surgery.
- Diagnosis.
- Equipment.
- Lab reports.

"They can happen during even the most routine tasks, such as when a hospital patient on a salt-free diet is given a high-salt meal.

"Most errors result from problems created by today's complex health care system. But errors also happen when doctors and their patients have problems communicating. For example, a recent study supported by the Agency for Healthcare Research and Quality (AHRQ) found that doctors often do not do enough to help their patients make informed decisions. Uninvolved and uninformed patients are less likely to accept the doctor's choice of treatment and less likely to do what they need to do to make the treatment work."

After disseminating useful life-saving information, they then told us that it's the consumer's sole responsibility to prevent medical errors. It's as if they were telling us, "We've been ordered to keep a low profile and do nothing, so now you all will have to save yourselves." Why have the members of congress been refusing to make health care providers accountable for prescribing the wrong medication, wrong dosages or multiple drugs that cause harm through unexpected chemical interaction? Why are they refusing to hold caregivers accountable for dilapidated equipment, lack of training, and wanton disregard for patient safety and well-being?

More than ten years after the Institute of Medicine came out with the revelation of 98,000 unnecessary hospital deaths per year, the industry and state governments have failed to protect us. Congress continues to refuse to address patient safety issues and medical errors remain behind veils of secrecy. Even protecting yourself has become impossible because consumers don't know when hospitals have an unsafe staffing level. They often falsely advertise that they will provide the best quality care knowing that they don't have the nursing staff or adequate supervision to live up to their false claims.

Following the Money

I had to wonder about the ten top companies that received a total of 632 million dollars in research grants for patient safety from 2000 to 2008. To justify the billion dollars paid out in total we should be able to find some expertise in patient safety.

First we have Westat, Inc. The services they advertise are study design and analysis developing statistical models, information technology and website design. There is nothing about patient safety in their brochures.

There was no need to invent new study models to know how many people died unexpectedly and what killed them. What in the world did they do for six years to justify paying them $363 million? Did the agency get a receipt at least? How many new statistical models did the tax payers get for a third of a billion dollars?

What if we had used that money to repair medical equipment in all of the public hospitals or to improve infection control monitoring procedures? How many lives could have been saved using those funds to actually improve the quality of care? These are the questions that a Senatorial investigation committee should be asking in a public hearing.

The second grant beneficiary was Social & Scientific Systems. Their principle business activities are supporting HIV/AIDS clinical trials around the world, providing program monitoring and evaluation services in Africa, collecting epidemiologic data in Europe, coordinating AIDS conferences in the Caribbean and Africa, and analyzing Medicare data in the United States. Their website has AHRQ at the top of their "largest client" list for $9 million that they have received annually for six years.

The third vendor of useless services is Research Triangle Institute. This is a think tank that provides research and development consulting services. They have one person, Barbara L. Massoudi, listed as an expert in health care quality and access, epidemiology, health information technology and health policy. Her credentials are in health informatics, environmental epidemiology and health care administration. There is no visible expertise in this company regarding medical error prevention or patient safety protocols.

The fourth federal fund rip-off recipient is the Emergency Care Research Institute (ECRI). Their mission statement says that they help health care organizations decide which medical procedures, devices, drugs, and processes are best, to improve patient care. Their decision paradigm is based on "evidence-based research."

This think tank is focused on which types of treatments can produce the best outcomes in improving the patients' clinical condition. According to their list of services, they also collect and analyze patient safety data and provide investigations of untoward events. Although this company's area of expertise seems to be related to patient safety at least in part, it is not clear exactly what services they delivered for the $31.5 million they received, other than more useless reports of unnecessary deaths for which the government response is to continue watching people die.

The fifth beneficiary of the political pork is the National Opinion Research Center of the University of Chicago. This think tank specializes in designing patient satisfaction surveys. Although there is some correlation between patient satisfaction and safety, why does it take $26.7 million to design and distribute patient satisfaction survey forms? I could have provided the same product and would have been happy for even one tenth that amount. Actually, I would have charged $2,000 for ten hours of work and could have given the AHRQ a very nice form covering all of the service points. If they wanted me to actually conduct patient satisfaction surveys across the board, I could have accomplished that project for a mere $150,000 over six years by distributing the forms to sample health care facilities, collecting them after completion and analyzing the results.

The fifth beneficiary of government waste is Thomson Company Inc. This is an engineering firm. They design high tech laboratory facilities for biosafety level 3. These are laboratories that work with lethal microbes for vaccine development and to develop defenses against biological weapons. This firm received $24.7 million for doing nothing.

The sixth lucky winner is Oregon Health & Science University. They received $24.6 million. At least they have schools of medicine and nursing and run a large hospital medical center. One would hope that they at least made some contribution to understanding how to prevent lethal medical errors, but we have not seen any government action arising from this service period of 2002-2008.

The seventh recipient of federal cash is Booz, Allen Hamilton to the tune of $24.2 million. It's not clear what they do specifically. Their mission statement is to help government agencies figure out what they're supposed to do. Perhaps they advised the AHRQ to give them 24 million dollars and keep a low profile.

The eight recipient of political payoff is Johns Hopkins University. Now, this is a fine institution, which is world famous in bringing about great advances in medical technology. I would be inclined to believe that giving those $23.4 million was money well spent, but we do not see any benefit regarding patient safety. This begs the question, "What did this fine institution do with the money that was allocated to finding patient safety solutions?

The last recipient on AHRQ's billion dollar money giveaway list is the famous Rand Corporation for the mere pittance of $16.8 million. Their mission statement is, "To help improve policy and decision making through research and analysis." They certainly have their cadre of health care policy wonks, but it's not clear as to what policies they recommended regarding patient safety.

In summary, the AHRQ spent one billion dollars in taxpayer money for high-tech research and analysis to develop a policy of keeping a low profile regarding patient safety. There have been no congressional hearings on patient safety despite the evidence garnered by the AHRQ and Obama continued the same policy of the two previous administrations.

Wrap up

Health care is a universal human need for which the demand is absolute, over which the suppliers maintain control. Doctors tell us what services and products to buy, in what quantities and when. Since the goal is to relieve suffering and survive, most of us are willing to pay anything to get it. The main problem is that most of us don't have the means to pay for health care when we need it. We have had to rely on third party payers for more than half a century. Therein lies the rub; third party payers, be they private corporations or State and Federal governments, have known for at least three decades that ultimately there would not be enough money in the entire United States to pay for health care products and services as the baby boomers become a population of senior citizens.

Therefore, as news of inferior quality of care in all health care facilities resulting in fatal mistakes became public starting in 1999, both the executive and legislative branches of government did nothing to improve patient safety. The systematic slaughter of 200,000 people per year became a non-issue. In short, the government spent more than a billion dollars over eleven years through the AHRQ to study the problem and watch two million people die. I used to think that the failure to institute patient safety standards was a result of stupidity, but now it's painfully obvious that the government considers such victims as expendable since most of them are senior citizens.

Finally, the cost of providing "anything goes" health care to all seniors over the age of 65 is so gargantuan that we are currently facing a $36 trillion debt that keeps growing by $26 billion per year. By the time the all baby boomers (all people born in the U.S. between 1945 and 1965) pass the age of 65, our society will not be able to pay for all of the life-sustaining treatments available and the economy will collapse, with no recovery in sight. The Patient Protection and Affordable Care Act of 2010 came from a government whose members had resolved to eliminating the high cost health care expenditures through a process called "preauthorization". People who need medical care to survive will have to call or write to request approval for any prescribed treatment and those answering the telephones from call centers in India or the Philippines will decide who shall live and who shall die.

2. Medical Mistakes
The Needle's in the Red Zone

During the first decade of the new millennium, we have seen a flurry of rhetoric coming from hospital public relations people about patient safety programs, yet after the federal government spent more than a billion dollars funding "patient safety research", the statistics kept getting worse. What's more, during the eight Bush years, Florida and several other states passed laws cutting attorneys' contingency fees by more than half on all medical malpractice cases. The same states passed laws requiring full disclosure of medical mistakes. No one thought to require full disclosure of dangerous conditions that increases the risk of falling victim to negligence, like a shortage of nursing staff, or equipment in disrepair.

Thus, in the final analysis, hospitalization keeps getting more and more risky and government policy makers remain aloof. Perhaps the ever increasing number of untimely deaths of senior victims who succumb to medical and nursing errors is a matter of convenience to the policy makers. What else could explain the persistent failure of government to establish safety standards? If the airline industry crashed an airplane every week, people would choose not to fly. Thus the public outcry would yield immediate action. On the other hand, when people have life-threatening emergencies, there is no other option but to go to a hospital. Also, everyone knows that his or her life will be in the hands of hospital personnel, so there is no public outcry; there is only an intense fear of imposing laws that are clearly in opposition to the expressed desires the American Medical Association (AMA). Thus we have yet to see the U.S. congress show any interest in legislating patient safety standards.

The Do-Nothing Patient Safety Law of 2005

According to the AHRQ bulletin dated June, 2008[8], "The Patient Safety and Quality Improvement Act of 2005 (Public Law 109-41), signed into law on July 29, 2005, was enacted in response to growing concern about patient safety in the United States and the Institute of Medicine's 1999 report, TO ERR IS HUMAN: BUILDING A SAFER HEALTH SYSTEM. The goal of the Act is to improve patient safety by encouraging voluntary and confidential reporting of events that adversely affect patients."

Congress took six years to enact a law in response to hundreds of thousands of preventable deaths per year that requires the government to study the problem and watch people die. By the time Congress enacted this law; 1.2 million people lost their lives to preventable adverse events in hospitals and rather than legislate patient safety standards they created patient safety organizations "to collect, aggregate, and analyze confidential information reported by health care providers."

Furthermore, AHRQ took another three years to post information about Public Law 109-41 on their website. They noted in their bulletin that many providers expressed concern that patient safety event reports could be used against them in medical malpractice cases or in disciplinary proceedings. They responded to this fear by reassuring the public that the Patient Safety Law gave privileged communication status to any information that a health care provider gives to report adverse

---

[8] AHRQ bulletin, June 2008 **http://www.ahrq.gov/qual/psoact.htm**

events, even to the extent that the information would be virtually inadmissible in a criminal negligence trial. In other words, a physician, nurse or allied professional can kill a patient because of a wanton disregard for his/her safety and well-being, submit a confession to AHRQ and this government agency would not disclose the evidence of criminal behavior to law enforcement; all for the sake of gathering information to formulate a new plan of no action.

The Universal Hospital/Medical Errors

The most astounding aspect of hospital mistakes is the commonality of them. We continue to see the same mishaps in different hospitals all over the United States. Thus, we must conclude that there is a major flaw in hospital design and health care methodology whereby there are conditions that lend themselves to acts of negligence. The key word is "avoidable". The hospital executives like to use the term "unfortunate but unavoidable" because it absolves the institution of liability. Therefore, in this chapter and in the two that follow, we shall examine some of the common hospital errors, their root causes and how the government planned not to avoid the "unavoidable." The health care system cannot protect you or your loved ones.

Errors of Commission: Overt acts that deviate from accepted standards of Care

Surgical Blunders

When a physician or other health care practitioner is performing an invasive procedure, there is no room for error. Yet, the human condition is such that people make mistakes regardless of how careful they may be. Surgery requires precision, timing, physical agility, split second assessment and responsive action. Even the most skilled professionals are not always at their best. There is always the possibility of an error in judgment and an unexpected complication. Additionally, the surgeon has complete autonomy; governed only by a vague standard of care, which is subject to interpretation.

    On the other hand, when it comes to the airline industry, the government imposes safety regulations to guard against pilot error. For example, such laws require that pilots must be well rested and sober for at least twenty-four hours before flight time. There are no such laws requiring the same safeguards for surgeons who are about to go into the operating room. The AMA has always lobbied against legislating patient safety standards, claiming that the medical profession has to regulate itself, because only doctors can assess the quality of medical services. Issues of public safety like a surgeon's sobriety, or having a steady hand and an alert mind don't receive any government scrutiny because the leaders of the AMA are against it. Of course, when a surgeon's physical and mental condition becomes unsafe, only the consumers are at risk; unlike pilots whose lives are also at risk. Hence, the doctors who run the residency programs usually force the physicians in training to work for 36 hours with no sleep. Consequently, most teaching hospitals use groggy, sleep deprived young men and women to perform surgery and other invasive procedures like inserting needles into spines and other parts of the body.

    Moreover, the bizarre government plan of no action in the face of such blatant public hazards remains a mystery unless one is willing to accept the possibility that government officials see the unexpected loss of life of senior citizens as a convenience.

We shall see in Part 2 of this book that the Patient Protection and Affordable Care Act of 2010 is the culmination of an insidious plot to reduce the population of baby boomers as they become eligible for Medicare and begin to require expensive services, equipment, supplies and drugs to stay alive. The spiraling costs with a tenfold increase in demand for high-end services over the next ten years will undoubtedly collapse the U.S. economy. The leaders of this country have apparently made a decision to sacrifice the senior citizens for the "greater good" by allowing the health care industry to lapse into a mediocre chaotic system that kills a portion of its consumers until it becomes ripe for a government takeover. Then the government will control the preauthorization process and be able to deny treatment for life threatening conditions with impunity.

To continue, surgery carries an inherent risk of death from infection, unexpected body responses, miscalculations, anesthesia mistakes, unforeseen drug reaction and uncontrolled hemorrhaging; and that's if the surgeons and their support personnel don't make any mistakes. If a slip-up occurs during, cutting, clamping, cauterizing, sawing bone, suturing and the like, severe damage can occur to vital organs causing permanent disability or death. The job of the surgeons is physically and mentally demanding. If they are not up to the task with their physical agility and mental functioning people die. I once worked with a surgeon who had recovered from a stroke. He had to ask me to close the clamps for him once he put them in place because his right hand was too weak to be able to carry out that task. He was owner of the hospital, so no one dared even hint that his surgical skill was compromised.

Traumatic Transfers

I have often participated in transferring patients from the operating table to a gurney. There is still no safe systematic way of doing this. The surgeons, scrub techs and circulating nurse gather the ends of a blanket that is underneath the patient and then "heave-ho" on the count of three. This method most often results in a traumatic transfer. Normally it wouldn't be a problem, but the people being moved have been cut open and sewn back together like garments. The slightest jolt could easily loosen a stitch that was holding a cut blood vessel, causing internal hemorrhage. The problem of post-operative bleeding from traumatic transfer can easily be eliminated with inexpensive hydraulic patient lifts. The AHRQ could have supplied every operating room in the country with a patient lift for a fraction of the more than one billion dollars they wasted on phony research

Trauma also occurs when nursing personnel drop people on the floor as they move patients from their beds to a gurney and back again. This happens when the nurses, aides or transport personnel forget to lock the wheel brakes. People also fall and sustain trauma when nursing personnel attempt transferring patients from bed to chair and vice versa, using improper technique. The use of a hydraulic patient lift device would virtually prevent every fall. Why do these careless mistakes continue happening? Why haven't the contracted researchers suggested buying gurneys with wheels that lock automatically when the gurney has stopped moving? Why won't the government provide financing for hydraulic patient lifts for every hospital and nursing home? One would think that for the hundreds of millions of dollars of tax payer money wasted every year, that there would be at least one patient safety expert with a "PhD" that could produce a simple idea for a solution to keep patients from literally falling through the "cracks".

Medication Errors

Medication administration, being a major responsibility of nurses, involves providing the patient with a substance prescribed and intended for the diagnosis, treatment, or prevention of a medical illness or condition. Any mistakes would cause serious complications including toxic overdose, adverse reactions and/or dying from an otherwise treatable condition. For adequate patient safety, nurses have to insure that they have the correct medication, dosage, time schedule, route of administration and patient identification. The number of mistakes that happen repeatedly in virtually all hospitals is staggering. A few institutions have installed electronic equipment to aid in reducing error, such as bar codes with hand held readers to match the unit dose with the patient, but these kinds of improvements are still too few to make a dent in substantially reducing medication errors across the board.

Additionally, the money wasted by AHRQ to "study" the problems could have gone a long way to finance the purchase of these life-saving devices. Thus, we have the technology to stop most medication errors from ever happening again and the executive branch of government through three administrations has made a decision not to use it, while financing bogus patient safety research.

Blood Transfusion Mismatch and Tainted Blood

The transfusion of blood and blood byproducts requires an exact type and cross match between donor and recipient. There are safety protocols that must be followed for each transfusion, which requires two registered nurses to check the serial numbers and blood type and sign-off on the verification ticket. Yet, with these safeguards in place, many people are still dying every day from transfusion reactions and contracting HIV and/or hepatitis from contaminated blood products. This is a clear indication that the safeguards are not working.

Furthermore, the Joint Commission on Accreditation of Health Care Organizations (JCAHO)[9] has reported that 10 out of every 12 blood transfusion errors end in death. The reasons they found for repetitive errors in mismatching blood types were lack of standard safety protocols, sloppy techniques and the failure to utilize state of the art equipment designed to eliminate most errors. The reason given for the tainted blood is the failure to screen out infected donors. A few hospitals have decreased their error rates by updating their protocols, but for the most part there are no standard rules and regulations in place to protect the public from transfusion related deaths. The practice of purchasing blood donations from indigent persons still prevails in many cities across the country. Despite the warning label that must be placed on the bag whenever the blood comes from a paid donor, most patients are not informed of this increased risk. With all the money that AHRQ spent on what was supposed to be patient safety research, why are there still no legal standards for patient safety?

Electric Shock

Patients suffer electrocution in hospitals when they are not being properly grounded in the operating room. In order to prevent death by hemorrhage during and after surgery, the

---

[9] http://www.jointcommission.org/SentinelEvents/SentinelEventAlert/sea_10.htm

surgeon must cauterize most bleeders during surgery using an electric cautery device that delivers 50,000 volts at the point of contact. If the patient is properly grounded, the cautery tip burns the flesh in a tightly controlled manner just enough to achieve hemostasis (no further loss of blood). If the patient is not grounded, the result is lethal electrocution of the patient and any operating room personnel whose is in direct or indirect contact with any part of the patient. Unfortunately, with about 96,000 surgeries being performed every day in the U.S., somebody always forgets to apply the ground pad or plug the wire into the cautery machine. I wonder if any of the PSO personnel thought of finding a cautery machine with a failsafe mechanism that will keep the machine disabled until someone plugs in the ground wire. One would think that there could be at least one life-saving idea for more than a billion dollars paid to 619 think tanks over six years.

Surgical Tools and Products Left behind

The operating room suite of any sizable hospital is like a refurbishing factory. There is a constant movement of dozens of people on gurneys in and out of this section of the hospital that makes the pre-op holding area look like a miniature bus depot. In each operation, there are hundreds of instruments, needles and gauze sponges in use and many of those items are placed deep inside the patient's cavity in the operative field. In every operating room the circulating nurse is required by state law to count all sponges, instruments and needles before the initial incision, just prior to closing the cavity and again while closing the skin. There must be a count sheet and that shows that every item that was put in the operative field is accounted for. If the surgeon left anything behind, then despite the fact that the nurse reported twice that count was correct, it was wrong. The surgeon screwed up because he or she was supposed to check inside with his hands to make certain that there are no foreign objects inside the patient and the nurse goofed because he or she reported that the count was correct.

This protocol is probably more subject to human error than any other hospital procedure because the counts are done manually in a high stress work environment. The surgeons often throw sponges and instruments off the field onto the floor to avoid contamination. The nurse has to find them and include them in the count. This problem can only be resolved with re-education of surgeons and their assistants. They need to be more cognizant of the need to keep all sponges, instruments and needles

Patient Falls

Falling is probably the most common cause of traumatic injury in healthcare facilities like hospitals, nurse homes and assisted living facilities. It is a common healthcare hazard. It happens so often in every hospital and nursing facility that filling out incident reports for a patient fall has become routine. The reality is that people occasionally fall wherever they are because of human error, medical condition, negligence or an inexplicable momentary loss of balance. The fact that we walk upright with the heaviest part of our bodies several feet from the ground makes us naturally susceptible to falling and awareness of this danger is usually not a part of our usual way of thinking.

Hence, since injury from falling in an institutional environment is not always the result of negligence, we shall review the standards of care related to identifying the risks and taking the appropriate action to prevent falls below in "Risks and

Root Causes." Seniors over the age of 65 are the most vulnerable age group. One of the most important functions in preventing falls is to assess the need for monitoring. Higher risk of falling requires more frequent observation. Surveillance technology is relatively inexpensive, so that there is no reason not to use AHRQ grant money to assist hospitals and nursing facilities in acquiring video monitoring equipment, unless the government prefers that people continue to suffer trauma and die from fractures and internal injuries.

Surgery Performed on the Wrong Body Part

Surgery performed on the wrong side of the body is a rare mistake, but it happens. It's not that surgeons would operate on the stomach when they are supposed to operate on the liver, unless they've got the wrong patient. However, when this mistake happens it would likely be mixing up right with left. We have two of almost everything; eyes, ears, lungs, kidneys, etc. Most surgeons will do a pre-op visit and draw a line on the skin at the place of the incision with a marker; the likelihood of such a goof is slim. Yet it happens and I saw it happen in front of me once when I worked as a circulating nurse in Chicago. The surgeon opened his patient's chest to remove part of the lung that had a malignant tumor. He opened the right side of the chest and found a healthy lung. The tumor was on the left side. This surgeon calmly closed the incision placed a chest tube and sent the patient to recovery. He then scheduled another operation for the following week to remove the lower lobe of the left lung. The result was an unnecessary scar and an extra week in the hospital with unnecessary pain. This surgeon however, was an honorable man, so he took responsibility and humbly apologized to the man and his wife. It was the first time in his illustrious career that he had made such a mistake and most probably the last. The patient and his family forgave the surgeon and there was no lawsuit. Human error is a fact of life and sometimes can cause catastrophic harm.

However, there is a simple way to virtually eliminate the possibility of such error by mandating the use of barcoded identification bracelets for surgical patients that state the type of operation and the body part. The circulating nurse can scan the barcode after placing the patient on the table and the computer can then read the information aloud through speakers just before the surgeon makes the initial cut to confirm that they have the right patient and are about perform the correct procedure on the right body part.

Surgery Performed on the Wrong Patient

Operating on the wrong patient means that the operating room nurse might have all the correct paper work but the two patients got mixed up in pre-op holding. When this happens there are automatically two wrong operations going on. In the operating room, where all customers are wearing identical gowns and caps they pretty much all look alike and they are usually snowed under with anesthetics before they reach the operating room. Sometimes there are two patients with similar appearance with the same last name, so the accidental swap happens. The barcode identifier would go a long way to eliminate this problem. Also, the circulating nurse should visit with the patient a day before, if possible, to gain some familiarity to prevent such identity confusion among the staff.

Wrong surgical procedure performed on a patient

Performing the wrong surgical procedure has more to do with the consent than anything else. The standard consent form allows the surgeon to do almost anything perceived as medically necessary once he or she has made the incision. However, the consent form should state exactly what the surgeon intends to do. Since the advent of diagnostic technology, exploratory surgery has become virtually obsolete so there is no longer any need for surgeons to have such wide latitude. There aren't as many surprises as there used to be, although there are times when unexpected anatomical structures present a challenge to achieving the surgical goal. The best way to alleviate the risk of having a surgeon perform unauthorized surgical procedures after the initial cut is to send a member of the surgical team to communicate with a designated health care proxy to get verbal permission after explaining the reason for the change of plan. Of course, there would have to be exemptions made for any life-threatening situation.

Excessive Blood Loss during an Operation

Surgery causes a lot of bleeding. The circulating nurse has the responsibility to estimate blood loss during surgery to avoid the complications of severe anemia. The procedure is tedious and inadequate. The nurse has to weigh the blood-soaked gauze sponges after retrieving them and add the estimated volume to the blood taken into a plastic container through the suction device. If the blood loss is excessive, the nurse has to report it to the surgeon and he/she must take action to replace the lost blood volume and cells to prevent shock and anemia. Apparently, this potential for lethal complication is too often overlooked. Post-operative anemia is insidious because insufficient red blood cells causes damage to the vital organs for lack of oxygen and nutrients. The only way to prevent this problem from recurring is to institute patient safety standards to define acceptable blood loss and require replacement therapy.

Circulatory Overload

Circulatory overload is too much fluid infused intravenously. The lungs fill up with water and the patient literally drowns from within and dies. This is a common error and it often happens as overcompensation when treating patients who go into shock. Careful measurement of intake and output is the key to preventing this lethal complication. There is no substitute for diligent nursing care in this matter. Measuring intake and output is a simple task. Figuring whether there has been a net gain or loss is matter of arithmetic. Yet this mistake keeps happening in every hospital because there are no patient safety standards with laws to hold people accountable for wanton negligence that causes death.

One physician, a gerontologist whom I interviewed, said that circulatory overload is a common complication in the treatment of elderly patients. For some unexplained reason physicians tend to be overly aggressive with intravenous fluid challenges when senior citizens go into shock from overwhelming infection.

Therefore, the solution to this ongoing problem is simple; a patient safety protocol to control fluid challenges to prevent pulmonary edema (swelling of the lungs). Why would our political leaders consistently refuse to take simple measures to prevent 200,000 deaths per year? Do they see this loss of life as a final solution to the out of control cost of health care for the elderly?

Contamination of Devices, Medication and Biological Materials

One of the most common and deadly hospital acquired infections occurs from the use of contaminated devices, drugs and biological materials. Many of the treatments provided in hospitals require the insertion of medical devices for monitoring and the injection of drugs. Those items all have to be handled with appropriate sterile technique to avoid introducing infection into the blood stream. Individual sterile technique is impossible to monitor. Doctors and nurses are using sterile injections and invasive devices multiples times every day, so no one can know when a contamination occurs. More than 100,000 people die in hospitals each year from infections acquired through such contamination. Most often the patient suddenly spikes a fever and a blood culture comes back positive. The cause of this lethal complication usually remains a mystery except for the fact that we know that there was a contamination of one or more of the invasive procedures or treatments.

The intervention for prevention would require technology that could detect when a sterile object becomes contaminated, educational reinforcement of sterile procedure protocols and video supervision of personnel engaged in handling sterile materials for corrective action. Again, the research funding activities of the AHRQ doesn't seem to support such goal oriented studies and the question remains; "Why?"

Off-Label use of Medical Devices

The Centers for Medicare and Medicaid Services has identified the deliberate use of medical devices for something other than for what it was intended as a significant cause of death or disability. The FDA approves medical devices for specific conditions or diseases and when doctors prescribe a device for something that was not included in the FDA approval, medical people call this "off-label use". The FDA has no authority to prevent physicians from prescribing or inserting a medical device for off-label use; they only have the power to prevent a manufacturer from advertising the item as being beneficial for any conditions other than those for which the device was approved based on clinical trials. Therefore, a doctor can legally prescribe a particular device for almost anything, unless such use is obviously life threatening. Certainly a doctor wouldn't be allowed to substitute laughing gas for oxygen. However, there are too many instances where doctors use medical devices for off-label use with no concern for the unintended consequences.

For example, one company called Medtronic, Inc. made stents to widen the bile ducts to allow freer flow of bile from the liver into the small intestines. There were so many doctors using this device to widen arteries in the torso and legs, that this off label-use constituted 90% of sales. The biliary stent was apparently causing a large number of injuries to the vascular systems of patients resulting in serious injuries. Orthopedic surgeons often use plates and screws that were designed for other parts of the body, with detrimental results. It seems that it would be a simple act for the government to bring this off-label prescribing under control.

Although it would certainly be counter-productive to prohibit such practices, it must be controlled. We need laws that will mandate that doctors justify their decisions to go "off-label." There must be some precedent for making such a clinical decision. As it stands now, physicians have a license to experiment. The AHRQ seems content to allow doctors to practice medicine by whim; "Let's try this and see if it works."

Air Embolism

Air embolism is a pocket of air in the veins through an intravenous line. The intravenous infusion apparatus is supposed to be a closed system with fluids only. However, air invariably gets into the tubing every time it is connected to a plastic bag of intravenous solution and most often the air bubbles flow into the veins. Therefore, we can expect air embolism to some degree with every intravenous insertion. This happens hundreds of thousands of times every day across the United States. For some bizarre reason nurse and doctors don't seem too concerned with this air bubble situation thinking that small amounts of air are innocuous. However, it's a fool's paradise because in reality, there is no way to measure the amount of air going in from the tubing and it only takes about 20 ml of air to cause lethal complications. While most of the air dissipates in the peripheral circulation before it reaches the heart, it only takes a tiny 0.5 ml air bubble entering the coronary arteries to cause cardiac arrest. Therefore, the entire cadre of nurses and doctors in the U.S. are not diligent enough to prevent the infusion of air bubbles into the patients' veins.

One way to prevent most of the air embolisms is to produce I.V. solution bags with the tubing already connected and primed. The other way is to infuse all intravenous solutions through an electronic pump that sounds off an alarm and stops pumping when there is air in the line. Such machines have existed for decades and have been grossly under-utilized.

Patient Suicide, or Attempted Suicide

Patients in psychiatric hospitals or in psychiatric units of medical centers have to go to regular hospital floors when they have physical ailments that need medical attention. Medical and surgical units are not equipped to handle psychotic patients. The nurses do not have adequate experience and training to deal with behavioral problems that can be extremely disruptive and pose a threat to other patients and staff. Patients who are on suicide watch are especially problematic. There is only one acceptable way of preventing suicide; one-to-one sitters that remain at arm's length at all times. There are no exceptions. If the nurse walks into a room and finds the patient hanging by the neck, had leaped out of the window, or with self-inflicted slash wounds, the death or injury is the result of gross negligence.

However, we don't have any legal patient safety standards to prevent such lapses in care. On way to resolve this problem is to have medical units within the psychiatric wing to handle intravenous infusions and other aspects of care within the controlled environment so that the staff is not overtaxed when required to maintain suicide watch or take other precautionary measures. Such solutions seem nowhere to be found in the AHRQ recommendations, and if there are any, no one seems to be acting on them.

Maternal Death or Injury in Low Risk Pregnancy

It is shocking that the United States Government should identify a repetitive problem of causing maternal death or injury during childbirth in a low risk pregnancy and not take corrective action to legislate patient safety standards. There is no explanation I can offer other than collateral damage in the decision to avoid preventing massive numbers of deaths in the elderly population. There would indeed be reason for suspicion if the government where to take aggressive corrective action to prevent fatal mistakes in younger populations and continue to do nothing for the baby boomers but watch them die.

There are standards of care, but there is no recourse against those who violate them. The key is the prompt recognition of late-developing life-threatening complications and decisive action in a timely manner. For example placenta privia, which is the separation of the placenta from the wall of the uterus, is one of the most frequent causes of late stage hemorrhage that threatens the mother's life. The health care system has the technology to detect early signs of such late-developing complications; however, even the most sophisticated technology is only as good as the people who use it. The labor and delivery nurses have the primary responsibility to monitor the condition of mother and child and report any changes to the obstetrician or nurse-midwife. Then the obstetrician has to be available to make the decision in a timely manner. When it comes to medical and nursing negligence, the lack of accountability is the chief enabler.

Newborn Death or Injury in Low Risk Pregnancy

When there are unattended birthing complications, babies are at risk as much, if not more than their mothers. I am reminded of a mother-baby malpractice case that I reviewed for a law firm. The mom was in labor for 11 hours after receiving Pitocin, a drug that intensifies uterine contractions. During this time the baby's heart rate went significantly both above and below the normal range. The doctor was off premises and the nurses didn't bother to report the fetal distress until after several similar episodes. The doctor decided to proceed with vaginal delivery and the infant's shoulder got stuck in the birth canal.

After being extracted with forceps, the child was born dead and had to be revived. The resuscitation was successful but the baby had severe irreversible brain damage. The child had suffered two strokes in utero on both sides of the brain, one being mild and causing no damage, and the second being severe and causing spastic paralysis over half of the body on the opposite side.

Clearly the obstetrician in this case violated the trust that his patient placed in him by having the mother go into labor under the influence of Pitocin without being in attendance. There is no way to prevent this dereliction of duty, because there is no way to hold anyone personally accountable. If the patient complained to the State Medical Board, it is unlikely that there would be any sanctions other than a reprimand. Many more patients would have to die or suffer disability before the State authority would launch any disciplinary action. The nurses also didn't have to face any corrective action by the nursing board and the hospital administration vehemently denied any wrong doing. Thus a newborn child has to spend a life time with severe disability because the doctor and nurses were in wanton disregard of their patients' safety and well-being. What's worse is that these "professionals" continue to practice in the same blasé manner with impunity.

Incompetent Spinal Manipulation Therapy

In today's health care systems, chiropractors perform a majority of the spinal manipulations. Osteopathic physicians (D.O.'s) and physical therapists also provide this service. It is usually done to relieve neck and back pain, although for chiropractors this is the primary treatment for a variety of existing and potential health problems. What is not so well known is the variety and frequency of adverse effects that occur when practitioners provide this treatment in a less than competent manner. The medical literature reports a number of complications such internal hemorrhage (dissection of the vertebral arteries), dural tear (outer membrane of the spinal cord), swelling, nerve injury, disc herniation, hematoma, bone fracture and stroke. Of these complications, the first is the most common[10, 11]. The symptoms are frequently life-threatening, and death occurs in some cases[12]. The actual statistics are unknown, but estimates in the literature state on average that about 30 percent of all patients treated suffer some level of injury and discomfort as a direct result of spinal manipulations. There is also much controversy as to whether there is any real beneficial effect from such treatments.

Regarding prevention, as long as we depend upon manual spinal manipulations, it is impossible to institute some type of systemic methodology to reduce the number of injuries or deaths. However, with non-surgical treatment of herniated discs, computer-guided intermittent spinal traction devices are now available in many spine treatment centers. This new technology looks promising as an alternative to manual manipulation, which is a crude form of traction, in reducing the number of injuries

---

[10] A J Barrett and A C Breen; "Adverse effects of spinal manipulation"; Journal of the Royal Society of Medicine; 2000 May; 93(5): 258–259.

[11] Johnson, Ian; "Adverse effects of spinal manipulation"; J R Soc. Med. 2007 October; 100(10): 444–445.

[12] Senstad, Ola DC; Leboeuf-Yde, Charlotte DC, MPH, PhD; Borchgrevink, Christian MD; "Frequency and Characteristics of Side Effects of Spinal Manipulative Therapy"; Spine: 15 February 1997, 22(4) Pp. 435-440.

and deaths associated with such treatment[13]. There needs to be more studies focused on this problem. One place to start would be to require informed consent whereby the patient and/or family members receive full disclosure of the inherent risk of disabling injury or death associated with spinal manipulation. This would undoubtedly prompt patients and providers to proceed more cautiously.

Patient Burns

People often sustain second and third degree burns while in the hospital. Most often, safety in preventing accidental burns is merely a matter of common sense. We don't need multimillion dollar studies to figure out how to set up burn prevention safety protocols. There are two types of burns that occur in health care institutions: thermal and chemical. The former usually happens when staff members spill hot drinks on patients or cause the patients to spill it on themselves. The prevention protocol is simple and cheap. Test the temperature of all liquids before giving them to the patients and never give liquid that is hot enough to cause burns. In fact, temperature testing should be the safety protocol for all treatments to avoid burning the patient with a hot compress or other type of heat application, like infrared massagers.

The chemical burns are nastier because they usually occur when a caustic intravenous infusion goes awry and leaks out of the veins, infiltrating the fatty and muscular tissue. The liquid burns the tissue internally and ultimately erupts into an open

---

[13] Alex Macario MD, MBA, Joseph V. Pergolizzi MD; "Systematic Literature Review of Spinal Decompression via Motorized Traction for Chronic Discogenic Low Back Pain"; Pain Practice 6(3) 171–178. September 2006.

ulceration damaging nerves, muscle, tendons and bone. The only way to avoid these types of negligent mishaps is to carefully watch the intravenous infusion and shut it off at the first sign of infiltration. It's impossible to avoid all infiltrations, but by frequent assessment, the nurse can minimize the damage.

One case in point regarding thermal burns was a nursing malpractice trial that I testified at as the patient's expert. This scenario underscores the all-too-often carelessness in hospitals and persistent refusal of hospital management to accept responsibility.

A young woman, aged 24, suffered second and third degree burns covering the sternum and upper abdomen (6% of the entire body) due to spilling scalding tea on her chest and abdomen while in the recovery room after undergoing a surgical procedure under general anesthesia. The Plaintiff contended that the attending nurse committed a negligent act by handing the patient a cup of scalding tea and walking away.

The Smorgasbord Defense:

Maybe the Plaintiff Lied About Where the Accident Took Place?

The defense attorney proposed multiple possibilities to explain away the burn and shift the liability to the realm of culpable negligence. First, since the evidence of the burn was indisputable, she suggested that the plaintiff burned herself after going home and made up the scalding tea scenario. However, this contention had no plausibility because the burn reaction of the patient's skin to the tea being spilled on her chest was a matter of record. The nurse noted redness on the area of the sternum and treated the patient with Silvadene Cream, which is a well-known topical medication used for severe burns.

Perhaps the Tea Wasn't that Hot?

For the second morsel in the smorgasbord defense, the defendant nurse testified that she cooled the tea with tap water before handing it to the patient, but admitted that she did not test the liquid to see if it was sufficiently cooled. However, she insisted that the tea was "warm and not scalding". This testimony was laughable because the forensic evidence established that the tea was hot enough to burn the patient and therefore was, by definition, "scalding hot". Furthermore, the defendant nurse testified under cross examination that it would have been a departure from good and accepted standards of nursing practice to hand a cup of scalding hot liquid to a patient in the recovery room under any circumstances.

If the Plaintiff Spilled the Tea on Herself, it's her Fault

In presenting the third defense theory of culpable negligence, the defense attorney argued that the patient was alert and oriented and therefore able to take responsibility for handling the tea without spilling it and burning herself. However, notwithstanding that the patient was fully responsive verbally; the record showed that the anesthesia was reversed only 25 minutes prior to the time that the nurses handed over the scalding tea. During my testimony I opined that appropriate verbal responses in a patient who is 25 minutes post anesthesia reversal is insufficient evidence of a full return of all mental faculties, coordination and fine motor skills. I testified that the standard of care is to not allow a same day surgery patient to leave the premises alone even four hours post reversal because there is a danger that the patients neuromuscular system might not have fully recovered.

The Hospitals Failure to Provide Necessary Equipment

Moreover, it was established from the record and testimony that the patient was sitting out of bed in an arm chair and that there was no bedside stand or over-bed table on which to rest the cup. As I stated in my direct opinion, this absence of any table or tray surface rendered the spillage more likely to occur and that the hospitals failure to provide such equipment was part of its liability.

In rebuttal, the defense attorney asked, "Mr. Sharon, is it fair to say that the plaintiff could have rested the cup on the arm of the chair while holding on to it?"

"Yes."

"Is it not also fair to say that if the cup had spilled over the tea would have spilled onto the floor?"

"The scalding tea could just as easily have spilled onto the patients lap." The jury returned a verdict for the plaintiff.

Misapplication of Restraints

The subject of restraints always comes up with the discussion of preventing falls in high-risk patients. There have been injuries related to the misuse of restraints including strangulation and loss of limbs. Falls and other injuries resulting from ripping out items such as urinary bladder catheters are also sometimes related to the failure to reapply restraints after removing them or to their improper application. To protect family and friends while in the hospital you need to learn about restraints and their appropriate use. The restraints currently in use are four side rails, vest restraints (e.g., Poseys), wrist restraints, and leg restraints.

Side Rails

Side rails are self-explanatory. Current standards require viewing side rails as a restraint because they restrict the patient's physical freedom. They can also play a role in causing injury when unattended elderly patients attempt to climb over them to get out of bed. Therefore, the training and education of nursing personnel must include the proper use of side rails, especially to avoid relying on them too heavily for fall prevention.

Vest Restraints

The vest restraint is mostly for elderly patients who are likely to attempt to get out of bed but are not constantly trying to do so. The proper application for most brands requires putting it on like donning a clothing vest and crisscrossing the ends at the front. The nurse then ties the straps together under the bed. All nursing personnel learn two overriding principles. Vest restraints are dangerous when not applied correctly or when used as a substitute for patient monitoring.

I have recently reviewed one case from the Southwest in which a nurse found an elderly male patient strangled in a vest restraint. The vest was on backward, which brought the neckline up to the patient's throat. The poor soul, while trying to wriggle out of it, virtually hanged himself. In many other cases, unmonitored patients had fallen on the floor or had wandered off while the vest remained on the bed still tied.

Wrist Restraints

Wrist restraints are for keeping the patient from pulling on intravenous lines and tubes. Such occurrences have disastrous effects, especially with lines that have been inserted into the chest wall. Bladder catheters have water-inflated balloons on the internal end to keep them from slipping out. When yanked out suddenly, they cause internal damage to the urinary sphincter. In men, the damage is much worse because the balloon is pulled internally through the length of the penis. So it is crucial to prevent this from occurring. The downside is that wrist restraints can also cause injury when not applied properly or the wrong type of material is used. Current regulations forbid the use of items like gauze rolls or orthopaedic stocking materials because they can cut off circulation and cause either nerve damage resulting in paralysis or gangrene resulting in amputation. The proper item is a wristband designed to maintain a comfortable space between the material and the skin and that remains in place with a Velcro fastener. The strap that restricts movement of the forearm ties to a loop that attaches to the wristband. Thus when patients pull on it (and they always do), they cannot cut off circulation to the hand. Most states have laws that prohibit the use of any other material.

Every hospital also has rules that require releasing the arms from restraints one at a time to allow full range of motion at least once every hour. Every nurse is required to maintain a restraint documentation record, and a doctor's order is required within one hour of the nurse's decision to apply such a measure. Hospitals also require that the doctors periodically renew and review such orders.

Leg Restraints

Leg restraints are the same shape as wrist restraints, only larger. Restraining all four limbs is only for extreme situations when dealing with a patient who is wildly combative. It is for short-term use only, and the same rules apply with regard to range of motion. To make sure that every limb receives full range of motion every hour, the nurse has to free one every fifteen minutes. In most such cases, the physician will order some form of sedation. When the medication takes effect, usually the nurse can remove the leg restraints.

Wrap Up

The truth is that the health care system is unsafe. The government will not protect you because the standing policy of both political parties is to pay hundreds of millions of dollars per year for patient safety research and accomplish nothing. The American Medical Association has seen to it that there would be no legislation to impose safety standards for hospitals and other health care facilities. Thus, the "standards of care" remains as a consensus within a particular health profession as to what a reasonable and prudent provider would do to obtain the best possible outcome. We have reviewed the common universal errors of commission that occur in hospitals and other health care settings. The government could put a stop to most of these fatal mistakes that take hundreds of thousands of lives year after year, but it won't. The only logical reason for this official depraved indifference to human life is that most of the victims are senior citizens because every preventable death will save the payer system from having to spend hundreds of thousands of dollars on future health care services and products.

3. The Never-Ending Story of Never Events

Errors of Omission: Failure to provide services resulting in an adverse event

This next discourse on medical errors has to do with many nurses and doctors basically not doing their jobs, which is to provide services utilizing the knowledge and skills acquired through education, training and experience. It is particularly troubling to realize that all too often doctors and nurses simply don't follow well established, evidence-based protocols to help people become well again. Most of the time it's a simple task being overlooked or remaining undone, with a treatable illness or injury ending in death or disability. The problem continues to escalate and simultaneously escape public attention.

Thus, it is difficult to understand this widespread inertia among health service providers. I have always approached my work with intense emotions, thinking *this person will die if I don't do my job right*. Of course, one can't survive too long with such a high level of stress, so there has to be some emotional detachment to remain objective. However, there also has to be some level of motivation, like some intense feeling over the fact that someone's life hangs in the balance. But people in health care continue to neglect their duties and the public seems oblivious to it. If Best Buy sold two hundred thousand computers that didn't work, there would be a public outcry that could put this retailer out of business along with the wholesalers and manufacturers. Thus, the absence of public indignation over paying for substandard services resulting in catastrophe is a phenomenon that requires some probative discussion.

Where is the Outrage?

According to the results of the Washington Post healthcare poll published on October 20, 2003, the public has been satisfied with the quality of the health care system today but worried about its future. The reported "deep anxiety" of individuals is apparently over being unable to afford access to health care in the years ahead.

The most common harmful acts of omission are neglect, failure to provide professional assessments, failure to follow established protocols and policies and failure to intervene with protective and preventive measures. Such oversights are occurring in every hospital from coast to coast with alarming regularity.

The poll in question noticeably unveiled a confounding absence of public outcry against so many unnecessary deaths and catastrophic injuries. Nonetheless, in our high-tech age of information infusion, one should conclude that the apparent lack of public attention does not necessarily translate to lack of awareness, which begs the question, "Where is the Outrage?" The answer is that feelings of fear and helplessness suppress the potential for outrage, causing people to live in denial. Most people know that if faced with a life-threatening condition their survival depends on the providers and administrators of emergency medical and hospital services. Therefore, the idea of calling them to task and demanding legislation to make people safer in hospitals and nursing facilities remains unthinkable.

On the other hand, the feelings of intimidation and vulnerability are nothing more than a story that has little to do with what happens. Ordinary people can easily learn the identity of the corporate directors and presiding health professionals who are in charge of making health care policy and hold them accountable for irresponsible behavior that compromises patient safety. Yet, the Department of Health and Human Services under the leadership of three different administrations over the last twelve years have refused to adopt a policy of enacting and enforcing reasonable standards of safety, which must invariably include checklists at the beginning of each shift, much the same way that pilots are required to go through their safety checks before each flight. Therefore, once again, we need to look past the veneer and realize that we are dealing with shadow government policy makers who view the systemic dereliction on the part of so many health care service providers as a convenient tool to assist in reducing the population of aging baby boomers.

1. Wrong Diagnosis due to Failure to take a proper history

In all clinical settings the medical and nursing histories are the single most essential component of the provider's initial encounter with a patient. Medical professors tell their students that the history is fifty percent of the diagnosis. The health care practitioner must get a story complete with a thorough description of the symptoms and their onset, prior history of illnesses, injuries, hospitalizations and surgeries. There must also be a family history to determine whether there is any possibility of hereditary predisposition to certain illnesses. There is also a vital need to know whether the person is allergic to any medications or food. The failure to take and record an adequate history leads to wrong diagnoses and ingestion of substances that can cause a lethal reaction. Hospitals and walk-in facilities need standardized forms that prompt the history taker to ask the right questions. Why didn't the Congress include legislation for such dire needs in 1,000 pages of law that carried "Patient Protection" in its title?

2. Failure to report changes in clinical condition

The nurse's primary duty in any hospital is to assess the patient's clinical condition at appropriate intervals and report any changes to the attending physician or the doctor on call. These observations are mostly about assessing the patient's response to treatment and are time sensitive. The appropriate frequency of assessment depends on the patient's condition. The more acutely ill a person is the more often the nurse has to observe for any changes. The failure to monitor clinical changes and report them is a rampant problem in hospitals and other inpatient facilities. As the workload increases for each nurse, more patients die unattended. The Healthgrades report of 2004 stated that the failure to respond to life-threatening conditions accounted for about 30% of the fatal hospital blunders. The ability to observe for clinical changes is the primary reason for staying in the hospital, so resolving the failure to monitor patients would have had the greatest impact in reducing preventable hospital deaths.

Hence the AHRQ could have easily funded surveys of nurses who are not working in hospitals to find out why. Based on the results of such surveys, the researchers could have devised incentive programs to attract more nurses to return to the hospital workforce. However, the executive plan of inaction prevailed, with tax payer money and human lives going to waste, again begging the question, "Why?"

3. Inappropriate use of Antibiotics

The failure to use antibiotics appropriately is a common error that boggles the mind. The standard protocols are simple and basic enough to teach them to first year medical and nursing students; namely, take a sample of the suspected infection source, run a culture and sensitivity test in the microbiology lab, and then provide one of the antibiotics to which the identified microorganism is susceptible. Unfortunately, many nurses and doctors still don't get it because we find all too often that the antibiotic prescribed is on the resistant list.

We also have a problem with doctors and nurses treating infection without obtaining a culture. Doctors often forget to write the order and nurses forget to remind the doctors that they cannot take a successful culture and sensitivity if they start the antibiotics first because the offending organism might be killed off to the extent of preventing its identification, only to have it return with a vengeance. Thus, it may seem that the doctor and nurses reached the treatment goal without identifying the pathogen, but there is more of a risk of the antibiotic not being effective, resulting in a new resistant strain, more virulent and harder to eradicate.

Furthermore, there is a problem with antibiotics not being given in a timely manner, which allows the bacteria to develop resistant offspring, given the adaption capabilities in generating offspring. Hence, we now find ourselves dealing with stubborn virulent infections like multidrug-resistant staphylococcus aureus (MRSA)[14], which are causing catastrophic illness and death.

4. **Failure to maintain safety protocols to prevent falling**

---

[14] MRSA is, by definition, any strain of Staphylococcus aureus bacteria that has developed resistance to beta-lactam antibiotics which include
the penicillins (methicillin, dicloxacillin, nafcillin, oxacillin, etc.) and
the cephalosporins. This infection is especially troublesome in hospitals where patients with open wounds, invasive devices and weakened immune **systems** are at greater risk of **infection** than the general public (http://en.wikipedia.org/wiki/Methicillin-resistant_Staphylococcus_aureus).

Falling is probably the most common cause of traumatic injury in healthcare facilities like hospitals, nurse homes and assisted living facilities. It is a common healthcare hazard. It happens so often in every hospital and nursing facility that filling out incident reports for a patient's fall has become routine. The reality is that people occasionally fall wherever they are because of human error, medical condition, negligence or an inexplicable momentary loss of balance. The fact that we walk upright with the heaviest part of our bodies several feet from the ground makes us naturally susceptible to falling and awareness of this danger is usually not a part of our usual way of thinking. Hence, since injury from falling in an institutional environment is not always the result of negligence, we shall review the standards of care related to identifying the risks and taking the appropriate action to prevent falls.

In a hospital or other inpatient facility, this innate human potential for falling looms large and must be a major part of every nurse's admission assessment. In fact the prudent nurse looks at every patient as having the potential for falling to the floor. The question as to whether a fall is preventable is a matter of degree of risk. The bottom line is that the only way to assure that any patient is not going to fall is for someone to remain at arm's length at all times. However, the indiscriminate application of such a level of service is impractical and must be reserved for high risk cases. Nonetheless, there are certain standards for ascertaining risk levels with the appropriate action for each. The basic risk criteria are as follows:

1. History of falling
2. Mental status, i.e. agitation, confusion, alcohol or drug intoxication;
3. Medical conditions such as diabetes, epilepsy, sudden drops

in blood pressure, heart block, vertigo, alcoholism, drug addiction etc.;
4. Bladder or bowel incontinence;
5. Environmental safety;
6. Availability of staff.

First, if there is a history of falling one need not go much further to identify a high risk. On the other hand, the nurse still needs to further evaluate the likelihood of recurrence and whether the danger is imminent or intermittent. It boils down to answering the question as to what prevention intervention is appropriate.

Second, the patient's mental status is a crucial element in determining whether there is an accident waiting to happen or is it reasonable to leave the patient alone for some period. The important step for the nurse is to think about what is likely to happen after he or she leaves the room. However, when a patient is found to be mentally competent, it is reasonable for the nurse to rely on that individual to take responsibility and exercise reasonable precaution like calling for assistance before attempting to get out of bed. Of course the call button must be within reach and there has to be a timely response as well.

Third, any medical problem that leaves open the possibility of passing out or losing one's balance is a high risk of falling. However, the more important consideration is whether the individual is going to attempt to get out of bed without assistance. Thus, once the potential for falling due to medical history is identified, the mental status and cognitive abilities come into play.

Fourth, the presence of incontinence raises the specter of risk because the presence of excrement in the bed or chair causes a person to become upset. There is often a strong desire to get away from the mess and the unfortunate individual steps onto a slippery floor in a state of agitation.

Fifth the environment has to be free of obstacles, so that the furniture must be arranged in a way that there is always a clear path to the restroom and hallway. Also, any spilled liquid or other floor hazard must be immediately removed.

Sixth, there has to be adequate staff to answer call bells in a timely manner and provide sufficient ongoing assessment. One of the primary functions of nursing is to continuously assess for changes in condition. With regard to fall prevention, each time the nurse sees a patient there must be another assessment related to fall prevention.

In conclusion, there is no substitute for attention. The question as to how much monitoring is required can only be answered on a per case basis. When a person is judged clinically to be a constant threat to self or others, then a one-to-one sitter remaining at arm's length from the patient at all times is necessary. If there is no constant threat but there is still a high risk, then the amount of monitoring must be established in accordance with the pattern of behavior. Sometimes once per hour is enough and sometimes a person needs to be watched continuously. Video monitoring is also a viable way of keeping a patient from harm as long as the nurses can respond quickly enough. The bottom line is that the nurse needs to keep in mind the patient's safety at all times. I have found that the most common mistake made in the assessment of fall risk is the evaluation of the patient's cognitive abilities. Finally, I have often discovered in my case evaluations that the nurse taught the patient about safety, got him or her to agree not to attempt to get out of bed without assistance, made certain the call bell was within reach and the patient got up and fell anyway. The problem stemmed from the nurse not taking into account the patient's cognitive ability and the capacity to comply with the instructions. The key word is reliability.

5. What to do About Restraint Safety

Restraints are sometimes necessary, but nurses must apply them only as a last resort. Nurses are obliged to closely monitor the situation and try all other means to maintain safety, including a one-to-one sitter. Family members can be extremely helpful if they have the time and dedication. If you discover that the nurses and doctors have placed your loved one in restraints, ask to review the pertinent policies and procedures, and check to see if the nurses are following them. Never presuppose that everyone is going to do what is required at all times. Reality just doesn't work that way.

Here is what you can do to assure that the restraints achieve the desired goal without accidental complications:
1. Ask the nurse to explain the rationale for using the restraints.
2. Ask for a copy of the written policy and procedure pertaining to the particular restraint being used.
3. Go over the requirements with the unit charge nurse.
4. Stay with the patient as much as possible.
5. Give frequent reassurance even if the patient does not appear to understand.

The health-care system cannot keep all patients safe from injurious accidents. New laws and regulations to implement improvements can help, but the only way to immediately ensure a safe hospital stay is for you, the consumer, to take control and safeguard yourself and your loved ones. You can do this as follows:
1. Demand the right to see all the care plans related to safety

and accident prevention.
2. Review those plans with the nurses.
3. Take the opportunity to voice approval or recommend alternatives.

The nurses should feel obliged to include the patients and significant others in establishing such plans of care.

4. Failure to provide and maintain pressure ulcer prevention

Bedsores (also called decubitus ulcers, pressure sores, or pressure ulcers) are the breakdown of skin resulting from excessive pressure that cuts off blood circulation. Friction burns also cause ulcerations when nursing personnel drag their patients on the sheets while pulling them up in bed. This subject deserves its own chapter because bedsores are one of the most common complications of hospitalization and exist in every hospital and nursing home.

According to the U.S. Federal Agency for Health Care Policy and Research (now the Agency for Healthcare Research and Quality), as of 1993, 10 percent of all hospital patients and 25 percent of all nursing home residents develop bedsores during their stay. Empirical data indicate that these percentages are on the rise. Bedsores are usually the result of institutional neglect, and although prevention is difficult, bedsores certainly can be prevented.

Skin ulcers develop from the weight of the body resting on certain areas of the skin for long periods and from unnecessary friction. A primary responsibility of nurses is to relieve that pressure of weight and to avoid the chafing that comes from dragging the patient's buttocks on the sheet. The fact that such a problem persists in every hospital and nursing home tells us that the nursing profession as a whole has not placed a high enough priority on maintaining skin integrity. To that extent, this particular aspect of nursing is an abject failure. Therefore, you will have to learn what duties nurses owe you and your loved ones so you can insist on those services.

My own mother's story illustrates this point and also demonstrates how some interference can really improve the quality of care you receive. My mother, at the age of ninety-one, was living independently. I was visiting her once or twice per week.

One day, about a day before my regular visit, my sister called to tell me that one of Mom's neighbors said she had not seen Mom for three days. Upon learning this, I called the hospital nearest her home and found out that she had had hip surgery because of a fall she'd taken while out walking. Although she gave my name and location to one of the social workers, no one from the hospital called me to tell me that she was there.

The surgery itself was flawless. Unfortunately, within two days after surgery, Mom developed a pressure ulcer on her tailbone (coccyx). Shortly after the doctor transferred her to the rehabilitation floor, the bedsore deteriorated from partial to full-thickness skin erosion (stage I to stage II).

I had asked the nurses repeatedly if she had any skin breakdown. They assured me that she was getting the necessary care and that her skin was fine. They either lied or really did not know about the wound until one of the doctors discovered it. I did not find out about it until the attending physician told me that he had called in a plastic surgeon for a consult to evaluate the bedsore. Even my mother didn't know about the wound until the doctor told her.

Feeling outraged that I had been misinformed; I went to the nursing office and complained to the supervisor. I asked if my mother had been identified as being at risk for bedsores. The supervisor said she would get back to me.

The next day I went back to the nursing office, and the same supervisor told me she had reviewed the chart and that the admitting nurse had identified her as being at risk.

"Was there a plan of prevention?"

"Yes. They were to turn her every two hours, improve her nutritional status, and keep her skin clean and dry."

"Did the nurses implement the plan?

"To be honest, the documentation leaves something to be desired.

"What's missing?"

"The turning every two hours was not fully documented."

"They left her unattended for several hours at a time, didn't they?"

"I cannot disprove that statement from the record."

"Wouldn't you agree that the presence of a pressure sore speaks for itself?"

"Yes."

"Nevertheless, I am now concerned with the fact that the wound deteriorated to stage II after she arrived in rehab. I want to know what your nurses are going to do about it. When I first asked them if my mother had any skin problems, they lied to me. Now I still cannot get a straight answer from anyone."

"I will ask the rehab nurse-manager to have a conference with you."

A few minutes later, the rehab nurse-manager came and invited me to his office. His first concern was to tell me that my mother had the bedsore when she arrived on his floor, so it wasn't their fault.

I told him that I was not interested in laying blame, but

since he brought it up; my mother's wound had gotten worse after she arrived on his floor. He asked me what I wanted, and I told him that I wanted to know their plan for treating my mother's stage II decubitus ulcer. I asked for an air-flotation mattress, instructions to the staff to turn her every two hours while she was in bed, and meticulous wound care. I also asked him to tell me everything else they intended to do to make sure this wound would not get any worse but instead would heal. He assured me that all the things that I requested were happening and were being documented.

The sad commentary is that in a hospital that enjoys a very fine reputation, my mother would have suffered further deterioration if I had not intervened with a complaint. I also fought for her to remain in the hospital when they wanted to send her out with the wound unresolved. As a result of my speaking to the nursing administration, discharge planner, and attending physicians about the liability they incurred allowing my mother to develop a bedsore, Mom remained there for an additional ten days until the wound healed.

However, in fairness to the nursing staff at this hospital, I must point out that once I brought the problem to their attention, the quality of care became exemplary. From this I learned (from the other side of the fence) that if you voice a legitimate complaint, nursing supervisors and staff would likely rise to the occasion and take immediate corrective measures. Conversely, if you say nothing, chances are one in ten in hospitals and one in four in nursing homes that you or your loved one will suffer the consequences of shameful negligence.

Bedsores may not sound serious, but the loss of skin integrity with even a slight break puts the patient on a slippery slope toward a painful course of deterioration and infection. The skin is a complex organ. One of its primary functions is to shield the rest of the body from a hostile outside world. Bacteria and viruses swarm all over its surface like an army of invaders looking for a breach in the defensive barriers. Once even the slightest breach occurs, the enemy invades and destroys without mercy. In such cases, the nurses, charged with preventing the breakdown, are like sentries who fall asleep at their posts.

The protective barrier function of the skin also works the other way. Thus an ulcer as well results in the loss of body fluids containing precious blood cells, protein, and minerals. The same breach that allows the enemy to invade causes the defending army to lose its weapons and ammunition. For that reason, the slightest skin break can be devastating to one for whom the stress of illness or injury has already strained the immune system.

The principle that I am clarifying here goes to the standard legal definition of the scope of practice of a registered nurse that you will find in every state and U.S. territory. "A registered nurse diagnoses and treats human responses to existing and potential health problems through such actions and interventions as health counseling, health teaching and actions restorative to life and well-being...."[15]

Accordingly, the responsibility of diagnosing the potential for pressure ulcers and providing preventive measures and daily follow up falls exclusively on the registered nurses. First, the admitting nurse must initially assess whether you or your loved one has any risk factors that predispose to pressure ulcers.

Second, the nurses must devise a nursing care plan

---

[15] New York Education Law, Section 169; the balance of this statute refers to administering physician-prescribed regimens and the prohibition against altering any existing course of medical treatment.

detailing what preventive action they and their subordinate staff (licensed practical nurses and nurse's aides) must take. If you find out there is a likelihood of forming pressure sores, you have a right to demand that the nurse show you or tell you what the plan is. Once you learn the one method of prevention that works, you will be able to assess whether the nursing care plan is adequate. Anything less is not acceptable because the appearance of even a small bedsore results in a high risk of infection.

Finally, the nurses must follow up daily and document the results of the protective measures. It only takes an hour for the skin to start breaking down. Therefore, early detection of prolonged pressure is paramount.

6. Hospital Acquired Infections: the Dirty Little Secrets

As stated by Healthgrades, Inc., hospitals actually kill 1 out of every 500 people admitted for inpatient services. The biggest culprit is hospital acquired infections, causing catastrophic illness to 2 million people per year and killing 100,000. That's about half of the all of the 200,000 deaths by hospital error. What's more is the bizarre fact that the hospitals were cashing in on all of this mayhem to the tune of a collective $27.5 billion in additional billing to third party and private payers. That's right; every time a hospital caused more illness or death it received a financial windfall. So our healthcare system had unwittingly created a financial incentive for complacency.

However, in 2008, the bureaucrats at CMS finally came upon the realization that hospitals were cashing in on their mistakes and issued a new Medicare reimbursement policy to deny payment for any additional length of stay brought about by preventable error, which includes all hospital acquired infections arising from contamination of invasive procedures and indwelling catheters. Thus the idea behind the new reimbursement policy is accountability. The message is clear, "We are no longer going to pay for your mistakes."

Moreover, the fascinating part of the new government policy is that such infections are now considered preventable whereas before the occurrence of infection was "unfortunate but unavoidable," notwithstanding the commonly known fact that most infections in the hospital are spread by the health care workers. They literally lift the germs off of one patient and carry them to others like so many flies, mosquitoes and rats. Thus, potentially, every hospital practitioner who touches a patient without first washing his or her hands will cause dozens of new infections every working day. Many victims succumb to this onslaught of thoughtlessness because they are already immune compromised. Furthermore, whenever there is a contamination occurring during an invasive procedure someone caused that contamination. There was either a breach of sterile technique, or the environment wasn't clean enough.

The fact that tens of thousands of knowledgeable medical personnel are wantonly killing about 80,000 people per year simple because they are too lazy to wash their hands and put on gloves is unconscionable. One way that government can bring this rampant pandemic under control is to force hospitals to publish their infection rates and face repercussions for making people sick. If any restaurant or hotel became a source of infectious outbreak, the local health department would shut it down within a few hours of the report and converge on the establishment to discover the source of infection. Why do hospitals get away with causing infections with such regularity that the consent forms have clauses saying that hospital acquired infections are an acceptable risk? Does this injustice exist because the elderly and highest-cost patients are the most vulnerable?

7. Failure to make risk assessments and a Workable Nursing Care Plan

With each of the known common dangerous complications of being in the hospital like infections, bedsores, falling, suicide and wandering off, the nurses owe their patients an absolute duty to assess the risk of occurrence of any of those. This falls within the scope of nursing practice as R.N.'s have the authority to diagnose potential as well as existing health problems. The nurse has to identify the likelihood of any of the aforementioned adverse events happening on his/her watch. Such assessment requires filling a few forms and calculating the level of risk. If the level requires preventive intervention, the nurse simply follows a predetermined protocol. The failure to provide this service has become seriously problematic and most often no one is even aware of it until the patient or family member files a lawsuit. While we have to expect that some errors of omission will occur, we are dealing with a systemic failure across the board in all hospitals.

For a solution, the only way to insure that all risk assessments are completed is to bring every hospital in the twenty first century with computerized charting. These health information systems have to be programmed to set off an alarm if any of the risk assessments and care plans remains blank for more than four hours after admission. I have worked with such systems and the possibility of error by omission is almost zero because the computer will prompt for entry and send a notification to the supervisor's terminal.

The U.S. News and World Report Hospital Survey: the Failure to Communicate

The U.S. News and World Report Hospital Survey Report (USNWR) had found its way a few times to the top ten hot topics of the day in "Google Trends". Although it's a good thing to have such openness about hospital mistakes that kill 200,000 people every year, we need to evaluate the criteria by which the good people of USNWR do their assessments. Therefore I have decided to respond to some of the sections of their methodology description.

USNWR: "The mission of the annual *U.S. News* Best Hospitals rankings has remained unchanged in 21 years: to help guide patients who need an unusually high level of hospital expertise. Other "best" lists factor in routine procedures such as hernia repair and unthreatening conditions such as mild heart failure. "Best Hospitals" judges medical centers on competence in complex, demanding situations, often with patients whose age or other health conditions pose their own risks. Replacing a heart valve in a man in his 90s, diagnosing and treating a brain tumor, and managing inflammatory bowel disease are a few of many examples."

Although judging hospitals as to how well they perform in critical risky situations seems like a good idea, there are some problems here. For one thing, there are too many confounding variables to make comparisons between hospitals regarding the death rates of patients with high risk conditions. For example if the researchers compare the survival rate of heart valve replacements of patients in their 90's the sample size would be too small to be of any statistical significance and the comparative analysis would have to take differences in pre-existing conditions into account.

USNWR: "For 2010-11, we ranked hospitals in 16

specialties, from **cancer** and **kidney disorders** to **orthopaedics and urology**. A total of 4,852 hospitals were put through our statistical wringer. This year, only 152 of the 4,852 hospitals evaluated performed well enough to rank in any specialty. And of the 152, just 14 qualified for a spot in the **Honour Roll** by ranking at or near the top in six or more specialties."

This is a telling statement about the quality of care in the U.S. provided that the surveyors looked at things like nurse-to-patient ratios and unexpected deaths and complications.

USNWR: "In 12 of the 16 specialties, hard data such as death rates, procedure volume, and balance of nurses and patients largely determined rank. In the four remaining specialties. i.e. ophthalmology, psychiatry, rehabilitation and rheumatology, hospitals were ranked on reputation alone; it makes no sense to take mortality data into account in specialties in which few patients die."

Excluding mortality data was a mistake since most of the deaths would be considered unexpected, requiring further investigation. The public would need to know which of those hospitals in which "few patients die" has the highest death rate.

USNWR: "Reputation (32.5 percent). Each year, 200 physicians per specialty are randomly selected and asked to list five hospitals they consider to be the best in their specialty for complex or difficult cases. The figure shown in the rankings is the total percentage of specialists in 2008, 2009, and 2010 who named the hospital."

Asking physicians to rate their hospitals is like asking chefs to rate the quality of food in their restaurants. The hospital performance is only as good as the physicians, nurses and allied professionals who provide the services. However, if you ask an off-duty nurse, you will most probably get an earful of complaints, and if you are doing a survey, it would be worth your while to listen.

USNWR: "Mortality index. A hospital's success at keeping patients alive was judged by comparing the number of Medicare inpatients with certain conditions who died within 30 days of admission in 2006, 2007, and 2008 with the number expected given the severity of their illness. An index number above 1.00 means the hospital did worse than expected and below 1.00 better than expected. Software used by many hospitals and researchers (3M Health Information Systems MS-DRG Grouper) made the severity adjustments."

The method of relying on the 3M MS-DRG Grouper is inaccurate at best. The severity scores in this software determine the amount of revenue that hospitals receive from Medicare and other third party payers. The problem is that the higher the severity, the more the reimbursement; therefore, hospital billing personnel tend to exaggerate the severity data as much as possible to enhance the institution's revenue. Consequently, since the actual severity would likely be less than what is in the 3M software reports, the "better-than-expected" death rate could be actually hiding a number of deaths due to negligence. Those hospitals that did worse than expected might only be guilty of having more integrity when entering diagnostic severity codes for billing.

In conclusion, it appears that the hospital ranking methodology is grossly unreliable. There is also the possibility that there may be some biases at work in naming the top hospitals. What's seems to be missing from the entire survey is an in-depth look at which hospitals are experiencing the largest numbers of never events, like death from narcotic overdose, choking, wrong surgery, surgical instruments and sponges left behind, traumatic injuries, bedsores, the percentage of hospital-acquired infections and the like. If the people in charge of the USNWR hospital survey want to get a reality check on which are the best hospitals, they should survey the nurses after guaranteeing anonymity.

Wrap Up

The public safety issue of hospital mistakes being the fifth leading cause of death in the United States has gained some notoriety, but the federal government's propaganda machine has managed to draw attention away from this real need for reform; leaving coverage issues looming large in the daily headlines. However, there does seem to be more chatter about it in the "blogosphere". It seems that since Medicare policy makers decided to refuse payment for medical and nursing blunders, all of the third party payers of health care services, such as state Medicaid systems and private carriers, have followed suit. On the surface, one might be glad of this change because until October, 2008, hospitals would actually cash in on substandard care. Hurting people was actually more profitable that healing them.

Although we can be certain that hospital executives for the most part were not making conscious decisions to allow untoward events to occur in order to increase their revenue, many have certainly demonstrated a lackluster motivation for taking effective preventive action. Therefore, it seems logical to assume that the prospect of eating the higher costs of hospital-induced complications would motivate the governing bodies to achieve a serious clinical transformation.

On the other hand, it is not so clear that the motivation

for denying payment for iatrogenic illness and injury is prevention for public safety. It seems more like a bandwagon that government agencies and insurance companies are jumping on to avoid paying large chunks of hospital bills. Moreover, in the new upcoming avalanche of payment denials, the third party payers will have to accuse the provider of negligence by identifying the unexpected complication as the result of a "never event" and satisfy the burden of proof against a vigorous defense. Each of these challenges will take more than a decade because of the several layers of administrative appeals that the parties must climb through before going to court. Therefore, it is more than likely that this new wave of financial pressure is going to be ineffectual.

Consequently, in order reduce the onslaught of wrongful death and catastrophic injury arising from hospitalization; we have to become more cognizant of the meaning of terms like "hospital mistakes" or "medical errors". We have to understand exactly what is going on in the hospitals that repeatedly cause the same blunders in every facility in America. The answer is clear; the physical structure, management style and method of delivery are similarly flawed, which causes the same mishaps to keep reoccurring. This situation is comparable to the defects in the Boeing 737 aircraft, which recently caused the cancelling of hundreds of commercial flights.

However, hospitals must remain open and financially viable to serve the greater good. For most families the hospital is an integral part of the survival of their loved ones. Therefore we need to understand the risks and root causes of these "never events" that are always happening, which we shall explore in the next Chapter.

4. Hospital Mistakes: the Root Causes and the Cures

Risk Factors

1. New Technology

Every time a newfangled medical device finds its way onto a hospital floor, somebody has to know how to use it. The usual types of gadgets utilized to assists in direct patient care are machines that monitor vital functions and those that deliver drugs and fluids into the body. Manufacturers always claim that their products are user friendly, but my experience has always been that if I don't read directions or get someone to show me how to use it, I would never be able to figure it out. Unfortunately there are too many nurses and technicians who try to use high-tech equipment without proper knowledge and cause harm to the patients.

One of the most common causes of hospital death is narcotic overdose via infusion pump. The system is called, "patient controlled analgesia" (PCA) which is an infusion pump with a button device that remains within the patient's reach. The nurse or physician has to program the pump to deliver a certain amount of narcotic each time the patient presses the button to relieve pain and set the maximum dosage. The idea is to allow the patient to access the narcotic at will but not allow more that the maximum dose that the physician prescribed. Unfortunately, nurses and doctors are making mistakes in setting the dosage limits and nurses are finding their patients dead from narcotic overdose.

2. The Teaching Hospital Dilemma

Teaching hospitals, as much as we need them, present us with a dilemma of having to bear the burden of increased risk of injury and death. Certainly, young medical school graduates must have a place to gain experience and learn their craft before gaining autonomy in offering their services to consumers. These places are called teaching hospitals and are always affiliated with or under the ownership of a Medical School. On the one hand, teaching hospitals are the places where people receive the benefits of the latest advances in medical technology and they serve the greater good by producing qualified physicians of all specialties.

On the other hand, those who run teaching hospitals are the antithesis of patient safety for two reasons. First, they force their residents (physicians in training) to work about 100 hours per week usually doing thirty-six hour shifts. Such residents often perform delicate invasive procedures after being awake for more than twenty-four hours. This has been an issue for decades and although there has been some progress in some cities like New York with more reasonable scheduling, the problem continues to persist.

Second, there is the issue of supervision when a medical student or intern performs an invasive procedure for the first time. Although the patients sign consent forms they are not normally informed of the fact that an inexperienced person is going to provide the service as a learning experience. Most patients of teaching hospitals are "service" patients, meaning that they don't have a private physician and have no coverage or are under Medicaid. This is mostly an uneducated population without knowledge of the fact that they are the unwitting "lab rats" for training physicians and trying out new methods and procedures to see if they work.

3. Nursing Staff Shortage

Notwithstanding the fact that a full staff is no guarantee against mistakes, an unsafe staffing level is the most visible indicator of general deterioration in the quality of care. The following is a short list of problems arising out of not having enough nurses on duty:
1. Patient calls for assistance remain unanswered;
2. Bedsores;
3. Medication errors;
4. Injuries from falling;
5. Failure to follow physicians orders;
6. Incompetent nursing care from lack of supervision;
7. Failure to report changes in clinical condition;
8. Narcotic overdose from patient controlled analgesia;
9. Fetal hypoxia[16] during childbirth.

The shortage of nursing personnel is a problem compounded by the fact that hospital administrators and nursing directors are not disclosing their unsafe staffing levels to the consumers. Therefore, hospital or skilled nursing facility advertisements stating that they provide the best quality of care in the midst of a nursing staff shortage are false. This policy of misleading the public begs the question, "Why do hospitals and other nursing facilities deserve our trust?" The answer is denial; because reality is unthinkable; to walk into a hospital for an elective procedure with full confidence based on false advertising and face being killed because there aren't enough nurses to respond in time to life-threatening emergencies. Thus, to think that we might be better off lying on a park bench rather than a

---

[16] lack of oxygen

hospital bed after surgery is more than we can accept. Since most of us don't know how to improve the situation, we simply choose to believe the propaganda.

Case in point: in 2001, there was a scandalous report of a man who had donated a portion of his liver for transplant into his brother in a world class medical center in New York City and died of neglect during the first night after the operation. The investigation revealed that he was hemorrhaging internally and the nurses didn't notice the drop in blood pressure and bloody dressings. At the press conference, the public relations person lied; saying, "This was an isolated incident and does not reflect the usual excellent quality provided by this fine institution. We have taken steps to assure that this type of mistake will not happen again." If this six-figure executive had told the truth he would have said, "This patient died of neglect because we don't have enough nurses to take care of all of our patients and we deliberately and shamelessly withheld that information from the patient and his family to deprive them of their right to watch over the safety and wellbeing of their loved-one."

4. High Patient Acuity and Nurse-to-Patient Ratios

The next two questions, regarding the nurse-to-patient ratio and the acuity of other patients who share the same nurse, will identify how much attention the patient is going to get. The nursing profession measures acuity in terms of how much assistance a person needs in carrying out activities of daily living, such as eating, toileting, and personal hygiene, and how much skilled nursing time is needed to provide medical treatments and medications. There are actually five levels in standard measurements of acuity that determine how many patients a nurse can reasonably handle, assuming all the patients are at the same level. The fact that on a typical floor nurses usually have a mixture of all levels complicates this calculation. Additionally, over the past two decades, patients have been surviving longer on life support, and their doctors are moving them out of the intensive care units onto regular floors, so you will find a larger of percentage of artificially ventilated people there. This formerly unacceptable practice has become a new standard.

At any rate, it is difficult to determine with any precision what an acceptable nurse-to-patient ratio should be because acuity can change drastically from one moment to the next. Nonetheless, in areas where nursing shortages are acute, the dangerous levels become obvious.

To simplify the discussion of acuity, I shall identify three general levels: high, medium, and low. High acuity would identify someone who is ventilator dependent with intravenous lines, drainage tubes, and/or catheters and who may require heart monitoring by telemetry or may have an open wound. Moreover, anyone who needs total care for activities of daily living (ADLs) falls in this category.

Medium acuity defines a person who has all or some of the lines and tubes of the high-acuity patient but is not life-support dependent and does not need the heart monitor. A patient with open wounds is also included. These folks would need partial assistance with ADLs.

Finally, low acuity pertains to those who are walking around and independent with ADLs. They only need minimal supervision, provision of medication and treatments, and teaching. Staffing levels in New York, Florida, Ohio, California, Texas, and South Carolina, to name a few states, have become dangerously low. It is common to find a floor with forty patients relying on three nurses where the acuity mix is 20 percent high, 60 percent medium, and 20 percent low. One would also find five or six life-support dependent individuals among the high-acuity group. This is dangerous, unacceptable, and commonplace. The irony is that through this threatening nursing shortage there is no shortage of nurses. There is only a shortage of nurses willing to work in hospitals. Considering their plight, this revelation should not astonish or astound anyone. Nurses work with their minds, their hearts, and their backs. They are accountable to a slew of bosses, regulators, doctors, patients, and family members in being required to anticipate and provide the needs of patients. The workload is often cruel, and there is the added pleasure of forced overtime turning an eight-hour shift into sixteen. At the end of the day, they have to worry about lawyers dragging them into court as defendants or non-party witnesses.

Generally speaking, these shortages have been running in cycles, since more than half the workforce are married women providing secondary family incomes. During prosperous times with less general unemployment, nurses leave the workforce in droves. During recessions with high unemployment, some nurses tend to come back. The difference now is that the baby boomers are getting older with no replacements, so the available human pool is shrinking. This, coupled with the fact that we baby boomers are also going to load up the hospitals as patients in the coming years, makes the future safety of hospital services look bleak with half the nurses and twice the number of patients.

There are both short and long-term solutions to these perils. The short-term resolution requires family participation. If your loved one is on a floor with three nurses, two nursing assistants, and forty-eight patients with the acuity mix as described previously, you have two choices. You can complain to the supervisor, or you can volunteer to participate in the care of the person for whom you are concerned. If you complain, the supervisor is likely to respond with, "I'm only a supervisor. I am not a magician." In reality, nursing supervisors spend most of their time finding nurses to work for the next shift because the prescheduled staffing levels are appallingly dangerous.

Thus if you volunteer, you will make a huge difference in keeping the patient out of harm's way. In tandem, the hospital management must do away with strict enforcement of visiting hours for family members who want to conduct a round-the-clock vigil to provide one-to-one care. Certainly, we have a right to expect full and safe service for the enormous amounts of money we pay for hospital coverage. However, the immediate concern is the safety of our family and close friends.

In the long term, solutions are also possible but more difficult. The relief of some of the endemic problems facing nurses in hospitals requires a willingness on the part of hospital executives to acknowledge that such problems exist. Then they need to look at options like nursing program scholarships and recruitment of foreign nurses. Regarding the latter, we need some changes in federal immigration law to streamline the process of granting work visas to registered nurses from certain English-speaking countries. There also has to be a more equitable distribution of the corporate revenue of hospitals. The chief executive who makes half a million dollars per year with a cadre of executives each drawing six-figure incomes cannot justify saying that the hospital is unable to pay recruitment fees and expenses to bring nurses in from other areas. Given the need for austerity, there should be a shift of some of the cash from executives' pockets to the cost of hiring and retaining more nurses.

5. Patients with Mental Status Deterioration

Patients with mental status deterioration present a high risk of injury and death because they engage in dangerous behaviors and require a higher level of attention for safety. Such patients require close and constant supervision to prevent injury and death. Being a nurse, I have seen every type of acting out behavior imaginable from mere forgetfulness to aggressive attempts at homicide. The problem of anticipating the dangers and controlling such behaviors lies in the lack of training and education of staff. Too many nurses on general medical floors usually don't know how to assess whether a person is likely to become a danger to self and/or others, or they simply fail to make such evaluations.

In the final analysis, the only way to minimize the risk of injury resulting from abhorrent behavior is to provide a one-to-one sitter. This is a person who sits with the patient at arm's length at all times. Some years ago, virtually every hospital had a cadre of volunteers called "candy stripers". Most of those young women were aspiring nurses who provided assistive care with feeding, bathing, toileting, mobility and emotional support. They were extremely helpful and now they are gone. Today, we face an ever increasing occurrence of "never events" that seem to be always happening. One of those hospital hazards is the danger of people falling and one of the main reasons why hospitals are unable to prevent these disastrous accidents is the lack of resources to plant a sitter within arm's reach of all patients at risk.

Therefore, I am proposing a solution that will allow hospital executives to alleviate the failure to hire sitters in sufficient numbers to protect the people who are likely to fall when no one is looking. There is an untapped source of free labor – every community has hundreds, if not thousands of people who need to perform a certain number of hours of community service. Every high school requires such activity for graduation and the judges of every court system impose mandatory community service as part or all of a sentence for various misdemeanors. Hence, it behooves all hospital executives to implement a program to recruit such individuals by contacting the courts and high schools and offering those people the opportunity to work as sitters to satisfy the mandate for community service hours. Nursing educators can train people to work as sitters for safety in four hours. Although there may be some concern about allowing people with criminal histories to work in a hospital, individuals in a court-ordered community service program are under a great deal of scrutiny and they are highly motivated to complete their hours without causing problems in order to stay out of jail.

In conclusion, this idea is a win-win scenario for all concerned because in the final analysis it is about saving lives. There is also the added bonus of teaching people how to care for and show love to a stranger who is coping with physical and emotional challenges and needs someone to watch over him or her like a guardian angel.

6. Staff Members in ill health

Since no sane person would want to be an airline passenger with a sick pilot at the controls, why would people want to put their lives in the hands of hospital personnel who are not well? Aside from spreading contagious disease to patients, nurses, physicians, therapists and technicians must be alert and physically fit while on the job or their patients suffer the consequences of poor performance.

Although there are some safeguards in the employment process to prevent hiring people whose condition would pose a health threat to patients, there are a number of deficiencies such ongoing health screening after hiring. There also needs to be better enforcement of preventing sick people from working. Hospital management often gives mixed messages between telling their employees to stay home if they're sick and imposing disciplinary measures against those who call in sick too often. It's a daunting task given the fact that an employer has the right to weed out malingerers.

7. Medical specialization: "It's not my job"

In the days of "Marcus Welby, M.D. (Circa 1960)," most people would have a family doctor who was usually a general practitioner and went to see a specialist for specific problems as new specialties developed. However, the age of medical specialization has come to the point that it actually increases the risk of death or severe injury. For example, a John Smith suffers a heart attack and the ambulance takes him to University Medical Center and after fourteen hours, the emergency room physician admits him. He has no private physician and is uninsured like 45 million of his fellow Americans so the emergency doctor has to admit John to Cardiology as a service patient.

Two days later, John develops severe lower back pain with blood in the urine, so the cardiology calls in the urology department to evaluate the symptoms and the resident's diagnosis is "kidney stones." One night there is a severe drop in blood pressure at 3:00 A.M. and the nurse calls the cardiology resident to come and evaluate the patient's condition. The cardiology guy tells the nurse to call the urology resident and goes back to sleep.

The urology guy says "Call cardiology" and hangs up. No one responds, so the nurse has to call the supervisor, who in-turn contacts the on-call administrator who gets internal medicine involved and by the time the medical intern shows up, the patient is dead.

8. Health Illiteracy and Poor Listening Skills; "What we have here is a failure to communicate."

The Institute of Medicine (IOM) Identified "Health Illiteracy" as a Root Cause of Medical Error and issued a report on April 8, 2004[17] stating that as many as 90 million American adults lack the reading and math skills needed to understand basic health information and navigate the U.S. healthcare system. The IOM identified a conceptual entity with their new title called "Health Literacy: a prescription to end confusion".

The IOM report specified that the list of skills required for a U.S. citizen to be health literate are reading, writing, listening, speaking, arithmetic, and conceptual knowledge. The IOM defined health literacy as "the degree to which individuals have the capacity to obtain, process, and understand basic information and services needed to make appropriate decisions regarding their health." At some point, most individuals – even the well-educated with strong reading and writing skills – encounter some health information regarding forms, a drug or a procedure that they don't understand. Aside from calling for the

---

[17] IOM Health Literacy: A Prescription to End Confusion (http://www.iom.edu/Reports/2004/Health-Literacy-A-Prescription-to-End-Confusion.aspx)

health care system to address the problem through improved health education, the IOM put the onus on physicians and other health care providers to listen to their patients to discern whether they have understood what they needed to know to participate in their disease management and/or improve their health status with preventive measures.

In my professional experience I have encountered thousands of patients in the home environment over two decades. Most of the people I interviewed who were on medications did not know the names of their drugs, or the potential side-effects. All they knew for the most part was the color, shape and what disease it was for (i.e. high blood pressure, diabetes, nervousness or infection)

There are two basic areas of concern in the IOM report. The first one is public awareness of where to go for which problems. This is a matter of public education and deals with the population before they enter the system and encounter a health provider. The second area of concern is the information provided by the physician or other health practitioner. This applies to individuals who are under the care of the particular health provider, be it a physician, nurse practitioner, chiropractor, H.M.O., home infusion company, etc. The IOM attributes the failure to ensure that patients understand enough to participate in their own care as a major cause of medical mistakes.

Therefore, part of the duty that a licensed health practitioner owes is to make certain that patient or responsible party understands the information that must be provided to the extent that the patient or significant other can participate in managing the illness and engage in preventive measures.

Case in point 1: in the first case, a man living in the USA who was not proficient in English received a prescription for

Tylenol with codeine. The label read: "1 or 2 tablets every 3 hours as needed for pain". The patient understood this to mean that he could take two tablets every 3 hours or more often as needed. He ended taking two tablets every hour until he collapsed from a narcotic overdose. He survived with a mild degree of anoxic encephalopathy (brain damage from lack of oxygen). The patient sued contending that it would have been a simple matter to ask the patient, "What is your understanding of the instruction regarding your pain pills?" and not doing so was unreasonable.

Although many would argue that people must take responsibility for misunderstanding simple directions, the IOM points out that approximately ninety million people in America are unable to understand medical directions as provided on labels, instructions and verbally. On the other hand, one can also argue that people know whether they understand something or not and if not, they still have the responsibility of asking for further explanation. However, the core of the problem in poor communication is not lack of understanding but misunderstanding. Health-illiterate patients most often walk away from a consultation not realizing that they have an erroneous set of instructions in mind that differs from what the health practitioner said.

Therefore, it is incumbent upon the health care provider to take a reasonable step to be certain that the patient received and understood the medical advice correctly. Additionally we need to take a look at the standard instructions such as "take one or two tablets every three hours as needed for pain" and perhaps change it to "take one or two tablets every three hours or less often as needed for pain."

Case in Point 2: the second case involves a 63-year-old man who was sent home from the hospital on intravenous

Morphine delivered via patient controlled analgesia (PCA). The man died of an overdose on the second day of the infusion despite the fact that his wife was checking on him frequently through the whole time. In the investigation that followed, it was apparent from the records that the home infusion intake nurse failed to provide sufficient teaching to the patient's wife. The wife simply looked at her husband, who was asleep most of the time, and thought he was okay because he was breathing and sleeping peacefully. She obviously did not possess enough health literacy to check for narcotic stupor by waking him up and seeing whether he was difficult to arouse. She needed to find out whether he could respond to voice, or required tactile or even painful stimulation to wake up. The nurse needed to make certain that the wife understood how to assess level of consciousness. It is likely that with a few extra moments of effective communication, the wife would have been able to know that her husband was in trouble and she would have dialled 911 soon enough to save his life.

9. Health Insurance: the Good, the Bad and the Fool's Paradise

The opening statement of the Obama/Biden Healthcare Reform Plan said, **"Health care costs are skyrocketing. Health insurance premiums have doubled in the last 8 years, rising 3.7 times faster than wages in the past 8 years, and increasing co-pays and deductibles threaten access to care. Many insurance plans cover only a limited number of doctors' visits or hospital days, exposing families to unlimited financial liability. Over half of all personal bankruptcies today are caused by medical bills. Lack of affordable health care is compounded by serious flaws in**

our health care delivery system. About 100,000 Americans die from medical errors in hospitals every year. One-quarter of all medical spending goes to administrative and overhead costs, and reliance on antiquated paper-based record and information systems needlessly increases these costs."

This political rhetoric about healthcare reform sounded promising even though access to health coverage seems more important to these people than preventing unnecessary deaths. Nonetheless, Obama's writers saw fit to mention the carnage from hospital mistakes. Although the 100,000 unnecessary death toll was understated by one half, one would think that even if we were to accept as accurate this 1999 estimate from the Harvard School of Public Health, the wrongful loss of life of one million Americans over the next decade would be the first concern on the minds of liberal politicians who professed to be so zealous for the well-being of us common folk. Even with this low-ball estimate, Obama could see that hospitals kill more people than terrorists. However, what we saw in the first paragraph of the Presidential Health Plan was that the rising cost of health insurance premiums got first billing. Perhaps this is so because the dead don't have to pay for health insurance. Is the loss of so many lives including 15,000 children per year merely coincidental, or is it the end result of health insurance company policies under shadow government support through three shifts of power between Republicans and Democrats?

In any case, it is interesting that the Obama administration had recognized that the health insurance industry was the underlying culprit in the whole health care debacle, like a colony of termites eating away at the wooden foundation until the house was ready to crumble. The most striking statistic was the doubling of premiums in eight years. Where did all that extra money go? Taking a look at the breakdown of national health expenditures in the U.S., between 1990 and 2004, we can see the shift in how the health care dollar had been distributed[18].

Hospital care expenditures saw a reduction from 35.1 % to 30.4 % while construction and capital equipment share fell from 5.3% to 4.6%. There was also a concomitant decrease in physician revenue share from 22.0% to 21.3% and the nursing home industry took a hit from 7.3% to 6.1%. On the other hand, the health maintenance organization (HMO) premiums went up from 5.5% of all money spent on health care to 7.3%. The other big gain in grabbing a bigger slice of the pie is the pharmaceutical revenue share going from 5.6% to 10%. What a shock!

Therefore, we can conclude that the shares of health care dollars are shifting more toward the 1000% profit for toxic drugs and HMO executive salaries and profits and less toward the provision of health care and investment in new construction and capital equipment. Furthermore, the piece of health care dollars for administrative salaries and profits had risen to 25%, which represents a whopping six fold increase in health dollar share.

In conclusion, if we are going to accomplish the stated goal of eliminating the wasteful spending we need to start where the health care buck stops – in the stakeholders' corporate pockets. We need to take the corporate culture of arrogance, incompetence and greed (AIG) out of health care and put administrative control into the hands of licensed professionals who will be held personally accountable for the quality of care they provide.

---

[18] http://www.healthguideusa.org

Wrap up

The poor quality of health care in hospitals and other nursing facilities is reaching critical mass. It's difficult to put a finger on the reasons, although it seems that the problem is in the programming. For example, my mother was once hospitalized for a fever. At age 96, that was cause for concern. While she was there I was able to prevent three major mistakes. The first one was a failure to order Digoxin .125 mg upon admission. This error occurred because my mom's regular doctor was out of town and the admitting physician didn't know her and didn't bother to inquire about her maintenance medication and the nurse didn't bother to tell him.

The second error was the attempt to give Mom an unnecessary bronchodilator respiratory treatment. The respiratory therapist came into the room and said, "I have a treatment for your mother." After I questioned the need for it, it turned out that the treatment was for another patient.

The third error was a failure on the part of the nurses to respond to my mother's call for help because she wanted to go to the bathroom. Fortunately I was there and went out to the nurses' station to find that some of the staff members were on break and others were doing paper work. They were completely oblivious to the call. I could tell that Mom, who was on fall precautions, was getting agitated and if not for my being there she would have fallen on the floor while attempting to get out of bed without help.

Moreover, of the three errors, the first and third would have had dire consequences. The standard of care with regard to medications taken at home requires that the admitting physician thoroughly review each medicine and decide whether to continue them or make some adjustments and it is a collaborative responsibility between the E.R. nurse and admitting physician. The standard of care with regard to the nurses answering the patients call for help is that the response time should never be more than three minutes with a patient who is known to be a fall risk. Otherwise, the probability of falling increases exponentially.

In conclusion, we know the root causes of the most common health care errors. The principle government agency in charge of patient safety, AHRQ was funded with over a billion dollars and accomplished nothing. More than two million people have lost their lives unnecessarily since the AHRQ has been in existence and over six million have suffered catastrophic injury. Congress passed the Patient Safety Act in 2005 which mandated funding a program of giving away tons of money and watching people die. Therefore the need for reform has nothing to do with access to health care; it has only to do with making health care safer and more responsive to our needs.

5. The Socialist Agenda and the AMA Capitulation

The White House Spin

President Obama originally outlined his overall agenda regarding health care reform with eight vague one-paragraph statements about what needed fixing. On the face of it, acknowledging that health care needs an overhaul and putting forth proposals for reform was the right thing to do. However, we need to smell what the politicians have been shoveling in our direction. When we look at the eight bullets of Obama's previously stated health care goals we can immediately see that patient safety and quality of care is near the bottom of the list as number 7 of 8 items.

Additionally, since health care blunders are the fifth leading cause of death in the United States today, we can see that in the Socialist-dominated government, saving money is more important that saving lives. Furthermore, when we analyze the eight so-called Obama principles as listed below and their order of priority we find statements that, while seemingly agreeable, offer clues that President Obama does not really understand the underlying problems which have a progressive history and root cause. Therefore I shall provide some in depth analysis of each of the eight "Obama" principles and point out where he needs to refocus his attention.

"1. Protect families' financial health. The plan must reduce the growing premiums and other costs American citizens and businesses pay for health care. People must be protected from bankruptcy due to catastrophic illness."

The word "premiums" is misleading because it denotes

that there is such a thing as health insurance. The truth is that health insurance per say doesn't exist anymore because the insurance industry has taken control of health care delivery. It started happening about thirty years ago with the introduction of the first pre-paid medical plans; Kaiser Permanente in California and HIP in New York and surrounding states. So, those families that have coverage fall prey to the policies of corporate HMO providers who save money by denying prescribed medical services, medicine, equipment and/or supplies for being medically unjustified. They also reduce cost by cheapening the quality of care being offered by discharging patients quicker and sicker from the hospital after teaching family members to perform skilled nursing services such as managing intravenous infusions and inserting urinary catheters. Therefore it is not the possibility of financial ruin that is the main problem; it is people dying or suffering terrible complications from treatable illnesses with the victims having no recourse.

"2. Make health coverage affordable. *The plan must reduce high administrative costs, unnecessary tests and services, waste and other inefficiencies that consume money with no added health benefits."*

While I agree with the statement, the term "coverage" is equally misleading in that the Insurance companies are not selling insurance anymore; they are selling a promise to provide health care as they deem necessary. The insurance carriers even have the power to override the treating physician's orders and if the patient dies or suffers permanent damage from a treatable condition after the denial, the insurance company and its medical review staff are immune from legal redress. Therefore, in order to reduce administrative costs while protecting people's lives, Congress will have to eliminate the process of precertification while enacting prohibitions against duplicating diagnostic tests by making the ordering physician financially liable for the cost.

3. Aim for universality. *The plan must put the United States on a clear path to cover all Americans.*

All Americans and non-Americans are already covered. Anyone walking into an emergency room anywhere in the United States must receive whatever emergency treatment and care that he or she needs to stay alive and prevent complications and the hospital personnel are not allowed to ask about immigration status. Then the Federal government reimburses the hospital for its bad debt losses. Consequently, the 46 million uninsured Americans plus another 30 million or so uninsured illegal aliens, including those who sneak across the border just to get free American health care, are using emergency rooms as clinics for most of the visits at $600 each. If we can move these people over to regular clinics and doctors' offices for $60 per visit we would save billions of dollars per year. Hence, it is not really a question of adding people to the health care systems; it's a question of providing the same care for one tenth of the cost.

Additionally, a big problem with talking about "uninsured" Americans is that the conversations always seem to exclude illegal aliens. Thus, we need to include them in all areas of health reform because they are entitled to health care under our laws and they have the right to sue for medical malpractice. Therefore, since the politicians and their advisers have been trying to make changes without factoring in the tens of millions of people who sneaked in across the Mexican and Canadian borders or the "tourists" who overstayed their visas, the entire effort will fail.

4. Provide portability of coverage. *People should not be locked into their job just to secure health coverage, and no American should be denied coverage because of pre-existing conditions.*

The customary practice of offering health benefits as part of an employee's compensation started with the rise of unions during the early part of the last century. This idea caught on as an important way to attract prospective employees. Now, everyone expects their employer to take care of their health needs. The other problem with an employer driven market is that HMO's offer different per member prices for different groups depending on the size and payout experience. This has resulted in price gouging the self-employed individuals and driving them to form associations to increase their buying power. It might be better for the economy to take the employer out of the equation and just have the employer supply all or part of the cost as part of the compensation package, but not be involved in the purchase. Then we could have all consumers buying health coverage on an equal playing field with diagnosis based exclusions being outlawed.

5. Guarantee choice. *The plan should provide Americans a choice of health plans and physicians. They should have the option of keeping their employer-based health plan.*

"Guarantee choice" is a popular buzz term to pander to the American consumer. The HMO's use it in their advertising to attract customers. It's effective because we Americans prize personal liberty above all else. It's a way of sugar coating nasty tasting medicine to get us to swallow it. The truth is that there is no such thing as freedom of choice in health care. As mentioned previously, this is the only industry where the supplier determines and controls the demand.

Moreover, when do we really have freedom of choice when we have no basis for making an informed decision? When we go to a doctor for the first time what information do we have about his/her track record? If you need surgery where can you go to find out that this surgeon performed that same procedure one hundred times before with forty patients improved or cured, twenty staying the same, thirty who got worse, and ten who died on the table? If I saw those numbers I'd be looking for another surgeon.

Furthermore, there are an alarming number of doctors and nurses who are being drug tested every week as a condition for keeping their licenses after being caught abusing narcotics. We do not know who or even how many because those records are not made public. Whether that would make any difference to you or not, by withholding that information the State licensing authorities are robbing you of your freedom to choose.

6. Invest in prevention and wellness. *The plan must invest in public health measures proven to reduce cost drivers in our system — such as obesity, sedentary lifestyles and smoking — as well as guarantee access to proven preventive treatments.*

The scary aspect of idea number six is that our government does not invest without taking control. Look what happened to the banks, Wall Street firms and AIG. The United States government now owns controlling interest of Citigroup, AIG, General Motors and a long list of other companies. So a government investment in prevention and wellness opens up a whole new paradigm in government playing a controlling role in our private lives. That is the socialist agenda. Socialism has always been about control of the masses for a few to have power. We need to understand that when we talk about preventive measures we are speaking of life style changes, not health care. Hence, in order to get people to change their daily routines to lose weight, the government backed new world order health plan will have to impose some sort of behavior modification on everyone who is over their ideal weight.

Additionally, we have all kinds of garbage food that we consume and feed to our kids that contribute to a high morbidity of chronic disease such as sugar, bleached flour, food dyes, preservatives and pesticides. Then there are all the environmental concerns like pollution and high voltage wires producing cancer-causing magnetic fields in populated areas. Finally there is just plain stress that is the biggest disease producer of them all. These are all areas that need attention, but do we want government to step in to impose behavior modification and start controlling the food supply?

7. Improve patient safety and quality care. *The plan must ensure the implementation of proven patient safety measures and provide incentives for changes in the delivery system to reduce unnecessary variability in patient care. It must support the widespread use of health information technology and the development of data on the effectiveness of medical interventions to improve the quality of care delivered.*

The idea of improving patient safety and quality of care should have been at the top of the list because of the fact that health care itself is a leading cause of death. If the government would focus on this problem, they could save about 200,000 lives per year and reduce the morbidity of another 300,000 or more. Since the same mistakes keep happening repeatedly in every health care facility in the country, there has to be something seriously wrong with the design and operation of every aspect of the health care system. It's like climbing aboard a defective airplane. For anyone who contracts H1N1 (Swine Flu), going to the hospital produces more risk of death than the virus.

Moreover, the government has already identified 28 events that occur in hospitals and nursing homes and will not pay for any care associated with those mishaps. We also know the root causes and what to do to fix the problems, with equipment changes, building renovations and professional re-education; this would take a large investment, but as long as Obama is throwing so much money around, it should be no problem to come up with a few billion to overhaul our health care. He can start with the VA hospitals and move from there.

8. Maintain long-term fiscal sustainability. *The plan must pay for itself by reducing the level of cost growth, improving productivity and dedicating additional sources of revenue.*

Making any venture pay for itself is a proper goal, but to what should we dedicate additional sources of revenue and where will all that extra money come from? In any event, we can achieve lower cost growth and improve productivity by simply making health care safer. The reduction in lawsuits alone would produce a huge savings as well as not having to treat preventable complications; and 100,000 more people per year alive and paying taxes would grow to a very large additional source of revenue.

Additionally, it is interesting that the American Medical Association, the long standing chief adversary of any type of socialized medicine and government imposed standards of care came out in support of Obama's eight principles of health care reform. The AMA has a well-known history of successfully lobbying against universal coverage. Consequently, the Congress excluded universal health coverage from the Social Security Act of the late 1930's and Harry Truman's health care reform efforts of the late 1940's fell apart in committee. Moreover, the AMA participated with the insurance lobby in slamming the door against universal health care coverage during the first three years of the Clinton administration.

However, since the Hillary Clinton fiasco, the AMA has done a complete 180 degree turn to the left and is now the biggest advocate for universal coverage. The explanation is simple; in the current world of Chaos, with the American and world economies still reeling from a state of collapse along with the hyperinflation of health plan prices, the physician customer base of health plan members and private payers is disintegrating. Thus the AMA sees health care reform via the socialist agenda as the only viable way to maintain their customer base and regain control of medical practice policies from the insurance companies.

The AMA Spin

In order to express this new policy of advocating universal coverage, the AMA sent a public letter to President Obama dated April 13, 2009 in support of his "Eight Principles of Health Care Reform". This may seem like good news on the surface, but if we unravel the spin and analyze each of the AMA's responses to Obama's eight principles we can see where this was all going and we begin to realize that the so-called health care reform as it has been formulated in Washington, D.C. is truly nothing more than adding politics to organized medicine to complete the world of Chaos.

April 13, 2009
The President
The White House
1600 Pennsylvania Avenue NW
Washington, DC 20500

Dear Mr. President:
"On behalf of the American Medical Association (AMA), we are writing to strongly support the eight principles for health system reform that you have set forth in

your Administration's budget. The AMA believes that we must enact comprehensive health system reform that will cover the uninsured, improve our healthcare delivery system, and place affordable, high quality care within reach of all Americans. We appreciate the opportunities we were given to participate in the White House fiscal and health summits as well as the meeting with physician leaders, and we commend your Administration on its extensive outreach to the physician community on health care reform. The AMA looks forward to continuing to work with you and the Congress as you develop health system reform policies in keeping with these eight principles. We would like to take this opportunity to outline our views on how to accomplish these goals."

What the AMA appeared to be saying without the spin: Thanks for letting us in on the deal, but since you politicians really don't know jack about how to deliver health care, we're going to tell you how reform it, but were not going to talk about how our mistakes, blunders and prescriptions are killing more people than most of the diseases we are treating.

"Principle One: Protect Families' Financial Health

"The AMA strongly agrees that any reform plan must reduce the rate of growth in premiums and health care costs so that patients can access the care they need. No family should have to file for bankruptcy due to exorbitant health care costs. The AMA supports insurance market reforms, such as protecting insured individuals from losing coverage or being singled out for premium increases due to changes in health status."

Without the spin: The HMO's are all done except for the ones that our members own and operate. We know we can no longer get away with charging those exorbitant fees that have bankrupted so many families, so we can blame the greedy insurance companies for the whole mess and shove them out of health care and back into selling subsidized insurance plans to every American.

"Principle Two: Make Health Coverage Affordable

"An examination of Medicare costs highlights the areas where we believe reforms can have the most impact in slowing the rate of growth in spending while simultaneously improving quality. Health care for just five percent of Medicare beneficiaries accounts for 43 percent of Medicare spending. The concentration of spending in patients with multiple chronic conditions shows where efforts should be focused to significantly improve the value that the nation gets for its health care dollars. Health care reforms should support efforts by physicians and other members of the health care team to better coordinate care and fill in the gaps in care that too often occur between hospitals and post-acute care providers. Access to better information through funding of comparative effectiveness research can also help bend the cost curve by supporting better decision-making by patients and physicians about diagnostic tests and treatment plans. The recent American Recovery and Reinvestment Act (ARRA) is an important down payment in that regard and we thank you for your leadership on this issue."

Without the spin: We're spending way too much money on old people with chronic diseases with forty-three percent of benefits going to five percent of Medicare recipients. Therefore, we can slow the growth of health care spending by withholding expensive high-tech life-prolonging treatment from the elderly who are going to die soon anyway. Thus, we should start making judgments on the quality of life and just throw people into hospice care if they don't meet our standards. Just give us the go ahead and we'll start pulling the plugs. Moreover, for those old folks who have trouble chewing and swallowing we can save tons of money by letting them starve to death rather than inserting stomach tubes for feeding. Oh, and regarding the recent American Recovery and Reinvestment Act, how about giving **us** some of that bail-out money?

*"**Through its impact on defensive medicine, liability pressure is also a major contributor to rising health care costs. Innovative approaches to reform such as health courts, early disclosure and compensation programs, administrative determination of compensation, and standards for expert witness qualifications could help reduce these costs.***

Without the spin: We couldn't resist this opportunity to blame the plaintiff lawyers for the fact that American health care is killing 200,000 people and injuring three times as many per year. Furthermore, since we are now in support of your socialist agenda, we intend to continue to refuse to accept responsibility for our negligent blunders, performing unnecessary surgery and taking bribes from pharmaceutical companies to prescribe toxic drugs for everything; including drugging children with amphetamines to control their behavior (to name a few). Therefore we want your Congress to give us our quid pro quo and protect us from having to answer to our victims in a court of law. Let's have health courts run by our members so that we can decide how much to compensate our victims, and set such standards for expert witness qualifications so that our victims would have to find doctors who would be willing to give up their medical careers in order to testify.

"The AMA also supports policies to make insurance coverage more affordable. Insurance market reforms and improvements, such as use of modified community rating, guaranteed renewability, and fewer benefit mandates, are needed to ensure that health insurance markets work better and rates become more affordable. Health insurance coverage for high-risk patients should be subsidized through direct means such as high-risk pools, reinsurance and risk adjustment. Premium subsidies and assistance with cost-sharing should also be available for low-income individuals who need financial assistance in order to afford health coverage. The AMA believes that the regressive employee tax exclusion for employer-sponsored health insurance should be eliminated or capped so that subsidies can be provided to those who need financial assistance in order to afford coverage."

Without the spin: when it comes to the insurance game we have no idea what we are talking about; but there are the high-risk groups like the elderly and we've got an aging population. Therefore, we'll have to add a high risk pool surcharge to the premiums. In other words, it's a big manure sandwich and all of the younger healthier people are going to have to take a bite so we can keep raking it in. Moreover, regarding tax exclusions for employer-sponsored health insurance, in keeping with your socialist agenda, let's finance universal coverage by taking some of the benefits away from people who work for a living and give it to those who don't. That way our member physicians won't have to reduce their income.

"Principle Three: Aim for Universality

"Covering the uninsured has been and continues to

The Socialist Agenda and the AMA Capitulation

be a top priority for the AMA. The AMA has longstanding policy to expand health insurance coverage and choices to all Americans, regardless of income or health status, and build on the current employer-based system to promote individual choice and ownership of health insurance.

Without the spin: Given the economic collapse and the massive loss of health coverage, health care as a business is in the toilet. So now we have to reverse our long standing stupid policy against universal coverage and throw in with your wonderful socialist agenda in order to keep our customer base intact so that our members can continue to thrive.

"The safety net provided by existing publicly financed health insurance programs (Medicare, Medicaid, CHIP, TRICARE and the VA) must be maintained and strengthened. We congratulate you on the passage of the Children's Health Insurance Reauthorization Act, a key first step. The AMA also supports simplifying the categorical eligibility structure of the Medicaid program to provide eligibility for all individuals with incomes below the federal poverty level."

Without the spin: As private health plans are being marginalized, you need to get Congress to beef up the reimbursement and let us take back control of utilization in publicly financed health insurance programs. Thank you for passing the Children's Health Insurance Reauthorization Act as a first step. Keep them coming.

"Principle Four: Provide Portability of Coverage and Principle Five: Guarantee Choice

"The AMA agrees that insurance must be portable and that individuals must have a choice among insurance options that best suit their needs. These are guiding

principles for the AMA's longstanding support for individually owned and selected health insurance. For those individuals who do not have access to or do not select employer-based insurance, the AMA supports establishing a health insurance purchasing exchange to increase choice, facilitate plan comparisons and streamline enrollment that will assist individuals in choosing coverage that best suits their needs. Insurers should provide information about their policies and costs to empower patients, employers, and other purchasers and consumers to make more informed decisions about plan choice."

Without the spin: as thousands of people lose their jobs we don't want them to lose their ability to pay for doctors' visits and hospital care. And let's do have a health insurance exchange for those who don't have access so we can get more "paid for" customers who can't complain because their getting it for free. Moreover, freedom of choice is a great sales gimmick because people will choose from a variety of plans on the insurance exchange that offer the same health care. Don't forget to keep in the co-pays and deductibles so we get keep on raking in some cash along with the capitation payments.

"Principle Six: Invest in Prevention and Wellness

"It is imperative that we invest in prevention and wellness to promote a healthy America. We will be unable to achieve the goals of improving quality of care and reducing the rate of growth in health care costs without such investments. Specifically, the AMA believes that insurance benefit designs should be aligned with current evidence on disease prevention. Public investments are needed in education, community projects and other initiatives that promote healthy choices.

Without the spin: we can afford to say we want to prevent illness even though we make all of our money treating it, because when you talk about investing in prevention and wellness, we know it's going to be a huge waste of money. Unless, of course, you plan on eliminating junk food, pesticides, air pollution, high voltage wires, poison chemicals, toxic drugs and stress. We also know that you can't measure prevention outcome. However, if prevention is what you want we can come up with a great plan.

"Principle Seven: Improve Patient Safety and Quality

"As leaders in the profession of medicine, the AMA shares with the Administration a sense of urgency and responsibility to meet the challenges that we face in creating a sustainable 21st century healthcare system. We are committed to creating a cultural transformation that better supports delivery of the highest quality care for individual patients and communities and which, among other strategies, will allow for a more appropriate allocation of finite resources. These two elements are extremely important, and we hold ourselves accountable to achieve them."

Without the spin: creating a cultural transformation is another way of making everybody think that we intend to change the way we practice medicine while we work on an elaborate scheme to have your Congress reallocate administrative costs and give it to the doctors. We are highly motivated in this endeavor.

"Health care delivery system reforms must empower physicians to improve health care quality and safety and make effective use of the nation's health care resources. The AMA believes that there are numerous reforms to the current delivery system that are necessary to provide

physicians and patients the tools to enhance value in our system."

Without the spin: Improve patient safety and quality? Bwa-ha-ha-ha-ha! Sure, just leave it to us. After all, Doctor knows best. You can trust us; didn't you ever watch "Marcus Welby, M.D.?" We just have to figure out how to improve on perfection. We'll just have to re-invent ourselves again with another new catch phrase.

"First, we must reduce fragmentation and improve care coordination with innovations like the medical home. New models such as accountable care organizations or incentive-based payments should be further developed and pilot tested before any widespread implementation. Further, through the development and use of care coordination measures, such as those being developed by the AMA-convened Physician Consortium for Performance Improvement®, we can begin to focus on those processes that produce better outcomes for patients and reduce fragmentation."

Without the spin: Reduce fragmentation and improve care coordination in the medical home! How's that for a new meaningless catch phrase? That is sure to impress your members of Congress. If "medical home" doesn't sound exciting enough what about dazzlers like "accountable care organizations" or "incentive-based payments"? You want us to be accountable for better care? Money talks! Just throw us a few extra billion dollars and our Physician Consortium for Performance Improvement will come up with even better ideas. We do great stand-up comedy too, but we're not kidding around.

"To encourage integration among physician practices we must remove legal barriers such as the existing

antitrust laws. We propose antitrust reform that would allow groups of physicians who certify that they are collaborating around health information technology and quality improvement initiatives to jointly contract with payers. Antitrust reform is critical to ensuring that the many physicians who practice in groups of eight physicians or fewer are able to participate in vital quality improvement initiatives that are facilitated by clinical integration."

Without the spin: Of course you will have to get your Congress to exempt all physician groups from the antitrust laws so that we can form a monopoly, engage in price fixing, punish any renegade physicians who won't join our organization and follow our rules and eliminate alternative medicines like acupuncture, chiropractics and homeopathy. Then we can have complete control over the entire health care industry, have access to all the newly digitized medical files of all Americans and form an alliance with the government health bureaucracies that will of course be under the President's control.

"Ongoing physician efforts to develop and implement clinical practice guidelines that promote appropriate utilization should be supported. Comparative utilization data should be provided to physicians and medical societies to help them manage finite resources. Further, physicians need access to patient-identified data on their own patients so they can improve care. We appeal to CMS to partner with us on new ways to share data with physicians to improve care."

Without the spin: Mr. President, to accomplish health care reform, you will need to issue an executive order directing the CMS follow our direction regarding clinical practice guidelines for appropriate utilization. They must give us access to all of their data and let us run the show.

"The AMA also supports the design of health information technology that provides relevant, actionable information to help physicians provide the best care, while providing the resources needed to employ these systems. The ARRA is a major leap forward by providing incentive payments for physicians who adopt HIT. We look forward to working with the Administration to ensure that physicians can adopt and sustain HIT systems and the quality improvement activities that they will enable."

Without the spin: We know the American Recovery and Reinvestment Act of 2009 (ARRA) set aside 20 billion dollars for Health Information Management (HIT) and we want that money! If you will grant us immunity from prosecution under the Antitrust Laws, we will be able to coerce most physicians to adopt and sustain the government HIT systems and enable the quality improvement activities that we dictate.

"Quality measurement programs must be truly focused on improving quality rather than solely designed for measurement or payment purposes. In the decade since the Institute of Medicine's groundbreaking report on patient safety and quality, we have moved beyond the "blame and shame" approach to try and foster development of whole systems that deliver safe, patient-centered, high-quality care. Programs that are simply designed to identify and penalize physicians whose results are below the top level of performance will not yield the system-wide improvements needed to assure high quality care for all."

Without the spin: Ten years after the embarrassing revelation by the Institute of Medicine that medical errors are the fifth leading cause of death in the United States, we have moved beyond the "blame and shame" approach because we refuse to accept any blame and have no shame. However, we did reinvent ourselves with new catch phrases like "whole systems that deliver safe, patient-centered, high quality care." This makes us look like we've actually done something to improve our services while the number of people killed by medical errors keeps growing. Therefore, rather than penalizing incompetent doctors for lousy performance, just grant us the power we are requesting with control of HIT and we will spin ourselves so clean that no one will even notice they exist.

"Health care quality data and measures also need to assess health disparities. Incentive programs must be carefully designed with adequate risk adjustment to avoid unintentional adverse consequences for patients based on age, race and ethnicity, sexual orientation, severity of illness, diagnosis, or economic and cultural characteristics."

Without the spin: We know that outcome incentive programs will motivate physicians to steer clear of sick people to maximize their good outcome statistics for the bonus money. This will also cause primary care doctors to avoid higher risk populations based on age, race, ethnicity and/or sexual orientation. Although we do favor such financial incentives, we have to be careful to appear as though we are eager to treat everybody.

Principle Eight: Maintain Long-Term Fiscal Sustainability

"The AMA has adopted many of the policies outlined above with the goal of improving care while ensuring long-term fiscal sustainability. In addition to these policies, the AMA believes that we must implement reforms of government insurance programs to ensure their

sustainability. Access to coverage does not guarantee access to health care services. Payment systems for physicians and other healthcare providers must be stable and adequate for the nation to keep its promise of access to care for current and future generations of senior citizens. We appreciate that the Administration's budget framework acknowledges that the threat of annual physician pay cuts must be removed."

Without the spin: We must have control over all reforms of government insurance programs to assure our sustainability. Remember, that you can have all the coverage in the world for everybody, but you can't have access to physician services unless we say so. Therefore if you want us to take care of the senior citizens you will have to return to paying exorbitant fees. Thanks for removing the annual physician pay cuts, but be advised that whatever you pay us will never be enough!

"We must explore new payment models and delivery reforms to address growth in health care costs and improve quality. The Medicare silos need to be broken down so that our elderly and disabled patients can benefit from an entire system of care that is organized around their health care needs rather than an arcane financing structure. Reforms should also provide appropriate incentives to patients by rationalizing cost-sharing."

Without the spin: On second thought, scrap the whole Medicare payment system, pay us what we think we deserve and if you go over your bloated budget, you can always increase co-payments or ration the care away from the elderly.

"In conclusion, the AMA looks forward to continuing to work with your Administration and the Congress as you develop health system reform policies in keeping with your eight principles. Thank you for your

strong leadership in this important endeavor."

Without the spin: In conclusion, you need our cooperation to make this reform scam work and we need your help to regain our former power and control. Therefore the AMA looks forward to continuing to work with your Administration and your Congress as you develop health system reform policies in keeping with our version of your eight principles. Oh dear leader, give us what we are demanding and we promise that we will deliver greater power into your hands with the entire physician community in support of your political agenda.

Wrap up

In summary, we can clearly see that the AMA leadership was blatantly vying for power and control and lobbying for enhanced income with immunity from prosecution under antitrust laws. While there is the need to take the management and financial control of individual medical practice away from insurance executives and give it back to the physicians, we also need to have standards of care imposed on them with accountability. However, the AMA was proposing to have Congress remove all accountability for negligence, eliminate physician discipline, put the CMS under their control and allow them to direct the implementation of all legislated health care reforms. There was not one word about protecting the public from the medical errors that have become the fifth leading cause of death in the United States. In view of the huge number of preventable deaths every year, with such a strangle hold on all forms of health care related activities, we seem to have more to fear from the AMA than the Islamic terrorists.

6. Medical Politics and Political Medicine

Recap

We've been had! Obama and his henchmen perpetrated a giant fraud on the American people and most of us never saw it coming. Those of us who were blogging away running up the red flags were just too few to have any meaningful voice. We have seen the culmination of a decades-old plan for the Federal Government to take control of health care and decide on who lives and who dies, with the ultimate ability to access health records on anyone and set up DNA profiles on every person. As we recap some of the political events since the Obama selection we shall see how this entire health care reform scam is solely about power and control and has nothing to do with improving quality and reducing costs.

Health Care Reform, Health Care Reform! Politics versus Reality

In the Obama presidential campaign of 2008, the rhetoric regarding health care seemed to focus on getting health insurance coverage for some 46 million people who couldn't afford the premiums. Providing emergency care for this population has always left hospitals with bad debt for emergency treatment. Of course, this problem put a strain on hospital cash flow and further deteriorated the quality of care. Add to that the millions of illegal aliens who have been converging on hospitals for emergency care and we have a more realistic picture of the financial meltdown that has plagued the hospital industry for decades. Even the federal funds that the Hill Burton Act has made available to close hospital deficits didn't do enough to stop many hospitals from going belly-up.

On the conservative side the presidential contender Senator John McCain proposed a five thousand dollar tax credit to the uninsured working poor and self-employed and told us to go out and buy a hospital coverage policy. That would not have worked because the cheapest family-plan price tag has risen to six thousand dollars per year and that comes with a deductible of equal amount. Thus, you would have to add one thousand to the government check and then pay out of pocket for the first six thousand dollars of health care costs anyway. This plan would have done nothing to help us stay healthy and treat relatively minor problems before they become catastrophic and there was no plan from the Republicans to protect us from medical mistakes. McCain's Republican proposal was nothing more than a shell game.

On the other hand, Obama said that he wanted to give us universal Medicare-type coverage but he didn't tell us how he intended to pay for it. Moreover, from the way things have been looking, Uncle Sam, with his raggedy clothes, has been holding his finger in the dyke while it's been collapsing around him. Thus, Obama's campaign teaser was a mirage.

What's important is what was missing from the conversations; the quality of health care. When the politicians said "health care reform" and talked about access, they were only displaying their ignorance. What McCain and Obama were not saying is that hospitalization itself has been the fifth leading cause of death in the United States. Hospitals kill more people than automobile accidents and some cancers. It's a paradox because we need hospitals to save lives, yet going through the doors significantly increases the risk of death or catastrophic injury for the survivors.

In conclusion, if politicians want to gain the confidence of the American voters, they need to level with us on all fronts. If they promise "health care reform", they need to be able to identify the problem and offer practical solutions, like an inexpensive way to provide clinical transformation in nursing by teaching them how to prevent the twenty-eight common "never-events" that seem to be always happening.

New Awareness of an Old Problem

The first major benefit of the Obama-Biden win was the new wave of news stories and commentaries on the subject of health care. This topic was rarely in the forefront and even during the campaign, it wasn't a major issue. However, now we began to see an amazing phenomenon; people were eager to talk about all the deficiencies in the health care system whereas before, the public consciousness was in denial out of fear of disturbing the status quo.

However, it seems that amid all this commotion about changing the way we do health care in America, our political leaders did not seem cognizant of what is really wrong with it. To accomplish this gargantuan task effectively, they first would have had to diagnose the problem with some degree of accuracy. To be sure, a universal health care plan to include the 46 million uninsured was a good concept. Still, the problem was much broader than lack of access for workers who make too much to qualify for Medicaid but don't earn enough to pay the price gouging HMO's. In fact, there have been so many things wrong with our health care; it was hard to know where to begin. However, we need to focus on some of the major issues like, poor quality, unethical practices, wasting financial resources, lack of accountability, and the drugs and Band-Aid culture.

First, when it comes to quality of health services, there is a legal concept called "the standard of care", which state laws vaguely define as providing services and/or making decisions with a level of competency that one could expect from a reasonable and prudent person of that profession. Thus, the health care professions and institutions are self-regulating for the most part and given that medical and nursing foul-ups have been a leading cause of death for more than a decade, our current system is an abject failure. Therefore, we need to develop standards of care for patient safety that specifies what a reasonable and prudent physician or nurse would do, such as take a thorough history, make timely observations, provide appropriate intervention in response to changes in clinical conditions and the like.

Although there are many who would argue against codifying standards of care, we need to take action to save two hundred thousand lives each year. There has to be more accountability. We can't continue to let people die in emergency waiting rooms while waiting twelve hours to see a doctor. We can't continue to allow people to develop bedsores because the hospital management won't provide a specialty bed and adequate staffing to turn the patient every two hours. We can't continue to allow doctors to give admitting orders over the telephone without ever having seen the patient; and we can't continue to allow hospitals to not warn their customers when staffing is unsafe.

Second, we need to put a stop to the blatant unethical practices on the part of health care managers. For example, the new reform plans should have prohibited hospital administrators from admitting patients beyond their bed capacities. Additionally, nursing executives who are usually aware of their staffing levels two months in advance, should have been required by law to report their anticipated shortages to the state regulators and be required to file a plan of correction within 48 hours of that report. The state regulators should have prohibited nurse managers from waiting until the prior shift before taking last minute action to alleviate the shortage by coercing nurses to work overtime. Such practices are commonplace and it has to stop.

Third, hospital board members should have been made accountable for fiscal policies that pay for elaborate parties, while patients fall out of bed because the directors won't allow hiring adequate personnel for patient safety. There has to be some control over allocation of financial resources to avoid leaving heart patients without proper cardiac monitoring, or leaving vital equipment in disrepair.

Fourth, we needed to hold decision makers accountable for the lives they ruin and the people they kill. The current system of hospital regulation allows for the levying of fines against the corporate entity. This system of adjudication is completely inane because it depletes the hospitals' financial resources thereby placing the patients at further risk while the individual culprits enjoy the protection of the corporate veil. The answer to this problem would be to require licensing of all hospital management personnel whose decisions have an impact upon the quality of health care services.

Finally, we need to change the mindset that health care is only about drugs and surgery. We need to demand the provision of health care from a holistic approach and mandate the recognition of viable health care alternatives. For example, instead of having a primary care provider deciding everything, we need a team approach with planning conferences that include the patient, who must have the right to approve the care plan or ask for another opinion. Furthermore, the patient should have the right to be informed of any legitimate alternative modalities.

To conclude, the fact that health care reform seemed to be foremost on the minds of lawmakers, the press and the public, was reason for cautious optimism. However, such hopefulness has turned to a sense of doom. While universal coverage under Federal Government control remains the ultimate goal, there is no one to take a deep look at the health care industry as a whole and call for congressional investigations into the reasons why there are so many unnecessary deaths and catastrophic injuries. What such congressional committees would uncover would be so shocking that new legislation would follow shortly thereafter.

Déjà vu

At the time of Obama's inauguration, the news media was all abuzz with health care reform rhetoric, seemingly waiting with baited breath for the unveiling of Obama's plan to make good on one of his big campaign promises, which reportedly was going to cost $15.5 billion. The Los Angeles Times reported that the Business Roundtable, the National Federation of Independent Businesses, AARP and the Service Employees International Union urged that a healthcare overhaul be a priority in the administration's first 100 days[19], but they hadn't said exactly what aspect of health care that they wanted overhauled. This ad hoc group intended to spend $1 million on advertising to keep the public eye on Obama in hopes of focusing the new President's attention on health care as a top national priority.

Additionally, the Business Roundtable expressed its

---

[19] http://www.latimes.com/news/nationworld/nation/la-na-health11-2008nov11,0,6833135.story

concern on health care cost inflation and lack of access due to an uninsured population of 46 million. The group's spokespersons stated that Obama made "health care reform" a major plank in his campaign but had yet to unveil what he is going to reform and how soon.

Moreover, other media journalists wrote that "health reform" was on the horizon. This entire barrage of media rhetoric begged the question, "What would Obama reform?" The two main concerns that public advocates and pundits were expressing were access to health care for the 46 million uninsured people and the ever-increasing costs. While those are important issues indeed, we had not seen or heard a single word about the ever-decreasing quality of health care services what with the nursing shortage, hospitals strapped for cash and doctors practicing defensive medicine. No one was paying attention to the fact that medical/nursing errors and hospital mistakes have been killing two hundred thousand people per year that we know of since we have been tracking this gloomy statistic for a little more than a decade.

Finally, after reviewing more than 200 news releases on this subject of health care reform, I have not found one word about reforming the way providers deliver their services to prevent so much tragedy; more than 2 million unnecessary deaths. It has been an unmitigated disaster and our government knowingly allows this carnage to continue unabated. We continued to relive the same tragic déjà vu moments; stuck in a never-ending loop.

Senator Baucus' Call to Action:

More Déjà Vu

Senator Max Baucus (D-Montana), Chairman of the Senate Finance Committee had publicly announced his intention to push congress into overhauling the nation's health care system during the first half of 2009. He, like Obama, wanted to force everybody to purchase health insurance once "affordable options" were available. Thus mostly high risk individuals would buy health care coverage causing the private insurance companies to abandon health care, leaving us with nothing other than the "public option." Once locking everyone into a single-payer government system, the Democratic Senator for Montana would institute "cost-saving focus on preventive care."

In retrospect, there were some serious problems with this not-so-new approach. First, there was no indication that this Senator or any other public official had any clue that the health care "system" was killing more people than most of the diseases and accidents. Regarding preventive medicine, it's great to give everyone access, but we have to have competent medical practitioners to do the preventing as well as adequate numbers of medical and nursing personnel to provide services in underserved areas, like rural and inner city communities and virtually every hospital in the country.

Second, the Baucus farce would have provided guaranteed free coverage for everyone living below the federal poverty line which would have included families of three making $17,500 or less per year. The rest of us would have had a federal mandate to buy a health plan in the "Insurance Exchange". This would leave the same gap that existed previously; people living somewhere between the poverty line and the point where they can afford to pay $6,000 per year for a health plan that has a $6,000 deductible (pay $6,000 in premiums and then pay out of pocket for the first $6,000 in health care costs). That group constitutes the 46 million folks who have never had health coverage. So, what did the good senator want to do, throw 46 million people in jail for not buying into the insurance company price-gouging swindle?

Third, if the Senator wanted to eliminate those crooked deductibles and lower the premiums, how would he have accomplished that? Was he going to force the insurance companies into insolvency and then bail them out like the corporate criminals at Fannie Mae, Freddy Mac, AIG, Goldman Sachs and all the other failed financial firms? Where will all that new money come from?

Fourth, the idea of affordable health insurance with no deductibles is something that we have all craved. However, we need leaders who intimately understand the practical every day workings of how providers administer health care in this country. At least Senator Baucus and Obama should have had better advisers to tell them that we needed re-education of nurses, physicians and other personnel, re-evaluation of the utilization of diagnostic technology, new laws mandating fiscal responsibility on the part of health care management, licensing of hospital administrators and a host of other specific reforms needed to turn political rhetoric into reality.

Fifth, the Senatorial call to action for health care reform in 2009 promised that once the government put the missing 46 million people back into the private fee-for-service health care system, they would improve quality and cut costs. Well, I have seen that same claim bandied about for the last 25 years with the introduction of managed care and prospective reimbursement. The cost cutting result was to push people out of the hospital quicker and sicker and deny approval for vital treatments.

In any event, if Senator Baucus and his colleagues were

truly going to roll up their sleeves and get down to unveiling a real reform this would have been a good first step. However, Senator Baucus proved himself to be nothing more than a political windbag in the middle of hatching the socialist agenda. Apparently, corporate executive accountability among health care organizations was never an issue because our leaders of the twenty-first century don't believe in command responsibility; we know that because they don't practice it. In the face of total economic collapse, we saw nothing but a lot of finger pointing with democrats blaming republicans and vice versa and no one made any moves to bring even one of the many corporate criminals to justice. What ever happened to Harry Truman's desk sign that says, "The buck stops here?" It got lost. No one saw it again after Nixon resigned. In the final analysis, what we really needed in health care is not reform but transformation.

Separating Fact from Fantasy

Certainly, it was encouraging to see Members of Congress, the President-Elect and the public take such a strong interest in health care. We had been waiting a long time for the cows to come home. Although Senator Baucus stated that his "Call to Action" was not a legislative proposal nor did it include all of the concerns that needed addressing, it did give us a clear insight as to how one of the most powerful persons in the Senate intended to approach the problem and solution as a whole.

Therefore, I shall present a careful examination of every statement and separate fact from fantasy, to understand that we should never have expected the Obama administration and his Congress to put forward any legislative action geared toward saving the lives of 200,000 innocent victims per year.

The Introduction

The introduction letter provided us with clues as to whether Senator Baucus did his homework in a way that empowered him to assess what was truly going on in the health care industry. If this was indeed a real call to action, then there was no more room for political correctness.

"In preparing to act, I led the U.S. Senate Finance Committee in holding nine hearings on health care reform this year and hosted a day-long health summit in June 2008 to explore in greater depth the problems plaguing our health system. I have spent a good deal of time talking to colleagues on both sides of the aisle and to stakeholders in the health care industry to get their perspectives on the issues that matter. And perhaps most importantly, in listening sessions across the state of Montana, I have heard from many Americans about the challenges so many patients and families face in getting access to affordable health coverage and paying medical bills."

First, it was good that the Senator held nine hearings and a day-long conference; but was that enough time to make an adequate assessment of a failed industry that represents one third of our Gross Domestic Product?

Second, it was not clear exactly who the "stakeholders" are, although in this context he is probably referring to people with a financial interest in the provision of health care services and products. However, the term "stakeholder" should apply to anyone who is affected by the outcome, which includes everybody.

Third, the people of Montana were not necessarily representative of the entire U.S. population. The health care experience varies greatly from one community to another. Thus, conversations with Montanans are only helpful with regard to Montana. Moreover it seems that what the Senator took from these conversations were complaints about lack of health insurance and paying medical bills. There was nothing said about quality.

"The plan outlined here addresses health care coverage, quality, and cost."

Coverage, quality and cost are the right issues to address but they are in the wrong order. Quality should have been the first priority because it is a matter of life and death. Medical mistakes are our worst enemy. Based on the number of domestic death casualties since September 11, 2001, we have much more to fear from our health care providers than we do the Al Qaida terrorists with the former causing about two million unnecessary deaths compared to about 5,000. Moreover, there is the bizarre fact that the greater harm comes from unintended consequences.

"The policies in this paper are designed so that after ten years the U.S. would spend no more on health care than is currently projected, but we would spend those resources more efficiently and would provide better-quality coverage to all Americans."

Again, the emphasis seems to be on cost and coverage. It would have been much more comforting if the Senator had said, "The policies in the paper are designed so that after ten years not one person will suffer unnecessary loss of life or catastrophic injury because of carelessness and stupidity."

"The health system is so complex that any solution will demand time and attention to make sure that we get it right. This plan is most certainly a work in progress. But this Call to action is intended to encourage constructive input by policymakers, stakeholders, and health policy

thought leaders to move us forward."

I emphatically agree with the complexity and the need to spend sufficient time and attention to "get it right". However, encouraging input from current "policy makers and policy thought leaders" was risky since this entire call to action was about cleaning up their mess. Regarding the "stakeholders", they will go along with anything to make a buck so we don't need to hear from them. We need fresh new ideas from people who have impeccable credentials as patient advocates.

The Real Story

To begin with, there was no valid argument against the statement, ". . . health care reform is an essential part of restoring America's overall economy and the finances of our working families. . ." The two trillion dollars that we have been spending on health care per year is twenty-five percent of our gross domestic product (GDP). Therefore, when the senator from Montana says, "Health care concerns are closely tied to economic anxiety," he was making an accurate assessment of the current public sentiment.

On the other hand, Senator Baucus stated that our big problem with health care has been lack of access and exorbitant cost with poor results prompting the need for better quality. I must take issue with his concern over the economic impact above the cost in human life and suffering as also indicated in this next quote: **"Each of these challenges has a direct effect on family budgets, on U.S. businesses, on government spending, and on the country's ability to compete globally. A better understanding of each of these key issues demonstrates the need for immediate action by the next Congress."**

Although I agree with this assessment of economic impact, what is conspicuously absent from the political rhetoric is the massive number of unnecessary deaths and injuries. This begs the question, "Why hasn't the mayhem of so many lives lost been enough to motivate congress to "take immediate action"? Of course, it is understood that the preventable deaths of parents, spouses and children generates such huge losses to our economy and society that we can't even begin to imagine. However, if we were going to be more effective in motivating lawmakers and their constituents to act, we needed to bring some unpleasant truths to the fore and say in loud clear voice that health care reform is foremost about saving lives! Certainly universal coverage has been a high priority, but if we don't immediately begin to identify the root causes of the same mistakes occurring repeatedly in every hospital across the United States, we will have universal coverage but we will miss the boat and millions more will die unnecessarily over the next ten years. This frightening prospect is what Senator Baucus and so many other leaders never seemed or didn't want to understand.

The Executive Summary

"**. . . Despite high levels of spending on health care, research documents poor quality of care received by patients in the U.S. Studies show, for example, that adults receive recommended care for many illnesses only 55 percent of the time. Children fare even worse. . .**"

The way the senatorial paper measured quality needs clarification. The example did not tell us why 45 percent of people with illnesses do not receive recommended treatments. If Congress is ever going to develop a workable plan, they need to have a clear concise definition of health care quality and know how to measure it. That actually is the whole point; to focus on quality first and then address the universal coverage issues.

Although I also am an advocate of universal health coverage, the lack of it does not mean that the uninsured are completely devoid of health care or are in a state of deterioration. However, even though we don't have any studies on the morbidity of this population, the lack of coverage does not necessarily preclude one from seeking help from a private doctor or engaging in activities that maintain good health. Moreover, with the internet and other technologies millions of people have moved into being self-employed and as non-group individuals, we left our group memberships behind and fell victim to the price gouging practices of hospitals, physician groups and HMO's.

Thus, for comprehensive coverage, solo entrepreneurs have to pay about $6,000 per year with a $6,000 deductible. For the average healthy person to pay that much to insure against a catastrophic illness and still have the pay the large deductible for various minor illnesses and injuries is beyond what most people can afford. Nonetheless, we need our congressional leaders to first focus on quality to save lives and how we measure quality is crucial to diagnosing deficiencies and providing solutions.

"The plan would refocus payment incentives toward quality and value. Today's payment systems reward providers for delivering more care rather than better care. A redefined health system would realign payment incentives toward improving the quality of care delivered to patients."

This assessment of physician incentives is not entirely correct. It depends on whether the primary care provider is on a fee for service or a per capita monthly maintenance fee with charge backs against the doctor for referring the patient to a specialist. The deterioration in quality occurred because of the policy of punishing doctors for recommending specialty care. This was an insidious method for reducing costs and caused a denial of patients' rights to competent specialty care because the PCP would make more stringent the criteria for specialist referrals. For example, the primary care physician, usually a family practitioner, who would normally refer patients over forty years of age with first time chest pain to a cardiologist for a stress test, would refrain from making many of those referrals after switching over to the per capita payment plan and provide the diagnostic and treatment services in-house. The PCP would then make the referral only if the symptoms persisted or worsened, and often the victimized patient would not see a cardiologist until after the first heart attack.

Apparently, the health plan moguls had adopted the policy of using financial incentives and coercion to control physician behavior to steer patients away from obtaining the vital treatment and specialty care for which they had already paid. The consequences of this scheme and others like requiring prior approval for all elective surgery and durable medical equipment were inordinate delays in surgery and specialty diagnostics causing millions of people to succumb to treatable illnesses. Therefore, we need immediate Congressional action to prohibit HMO's or any other corporate controlling entity from interfering with or attempting to change a legally prescribed medical regimen; and to prohibit all provisions in health plan contracts requiring prior approval for any legally prescribed medical treatment or surgical intervention.

The Political Plan: "Improving Value by Reforming the

Health Care Delivery System"

It's nice that Senator Baucus and his colleagues wanted to improve value, or get more bang for the buck by reforming the "health care delivery system." However, the term itself is an oxymoron because the word system denotes organization with one mind and purpose. The ironic truth is that not only is there no "system" as such, but the deadly mistakes are systematic in that they occur repeatedly in every hospital across America. Aside from killing 23 people every hour by negligence, hospitals do not do anything systematically. Each facility can create its own policy, which is often in direct violation of fire codes and health department regulations. There are no codified ethical standards for implementing hospital management policy. Thus, you can't reform the "health care delivery system" because it does not exist.

Therefore, congress needs to create a real health care delivery system that by law would require hospital management personnel and health care professionals to conform to certain standards of ethics and human decency, which should include, but is not limited to, the following:

1. All equipment must be in good working order;
2. Buildings must conform to fire and safety codes;
3. All professional personnel files must be in compliance at all times;
4. Safe nurse-to-patient ratios must be established by federal statute;
5. All units must conform to safe staffing ratios;
6. Every patient unit in the emergency department must have a cardiac monitor, oxygen delivery system and suction in good working order;
7. All supplies required for nursing care must be on hand;
8. All architectural designs for any new construction or

renovation of any hospital or nursing facility must have Registered Nurse approval;
9. All staffing coordinators must submit a staffing schedule two months in advance and report any shortfalls to the health department or other regulating authority and the hospital must submit a plan for obtaining the required number of nursing staff;
10. All hospital administrators must put their emergency departments on diversion when all inpatient beds are occupied;
11. It must be forbidden for hospitals to house patients in the emergency department for more than four hours after admission while waiting for an available bed;
12. Nurses must immediately report adverse changes in clinical condition to the attending physician.
13. Nurses must provide risk assessment for falling;
14. Nurses must provide risk assessment for bedsores;
15. Hospital management must inform the family members or significant others when the patient is at risk for falls or bedsores and present the plan of care for prevention;
16. Patients or their advocates must have the right to appeal if they are not satisfied with the plan for prevention of falls and bedsores;
17. There must be a law to forbid drawing more blood for testing than is required to actually perform the test;
18. Hospital management must have adequate personnel for sitting with patients to prevent falling and other traumatic injuries;
19. Nurse must turn all patients at risk for bedsores every two hours and the hospital must provide a specialty bed.
20. Nurse must respond at least by intercom system to a patient's

call for help within three minutes.
21. All patients must be within earshot of a nurse's station (place where nurses sit down to write their notes, make phone calls and review charts) and all patient units must be video monitored.
22. All personnel must wash hands with antiseptic soap before any hands on patient contact;
23. All isolation protocols must be adhered to.

In conclusion, we can see clearly that Senator Baucus and his Congressional colleagues either did not know what has been really going on in health care or never wanted to know. In any event, as mentioned previously, they can't reform what doesn't exist. They have to build a system of health care from the ground up by imposing the above standards and making hospital managers personally accountable for violations. The bad practices alluded to above are wantonly dangerous and commonplace.

Wrap Up

We can now begin to see how Obama, who started his presidency with a powerful control over both houses of Congress, has sucked us into a false debate over how to fix a "broken" health care system. Baucus, the lead dog in the Senate spearheaded the political rhetoric about the dire need for reforms making access to coverage, cutting costs and improving quality the primary issues with no mention of patient safety. Then certain leaders in the private sector of the health care industry chimed in with a phony new buzzword; "patient centered medical home." Reading between the lines, the HMO's were initiating program of total control over health care decisions with no alternative treatment options, while serving milk and cookies in a homey environment.

As we evaluate how we arrived at the passing of the convoluted Patient Protection and Affordable Care Act in March 2010, we can begin to understand American politics in action. It's about pushing an agenda of power and control with elaborate schemes and brazen behavior that left most people bewildered and stunned. The "new wave" politicians in Washington have sunk to a new low that makes Tammany Hall look like a bastion of holiness.

7. Healthcare Reform: First do no Harm

There is an old story from the bible that is not so well known, but it's there; it's about the leviathan. G-d created both the male and the female of this gargantuan sea dweller, but kept them apart placing the female in the spiritual world by killing it and leaving the male at the bottom of the oceans. The Almighty kept them from mating because if they had offspring, there would have been no room left on the planet for anyone else. So now, this leviathan stays at the bottom of all of the oceans (being that he is so large he has to stay wrapped around the entire planet). Thus, he just lays there eating tons of fish every day and if he were to raise his head, the tidal wave would wipe out the coastal areas on both sides of whichever ocean his head is at the bottom of. Well, health care in the United States is the leviathan in the U.S. economic ocean and it is getting very restless.

In other words, our society has created a monster that is killing 200,000 people every year while sucking in our money like a giant vacuum cleaner and we just can't afford to feed it anymore. It has grown so large that it takes up a third of the economy. If it hiccups, burps or passes wind the tidal wave would send us reeling and make the bank collapse look like prosperity. So what do we do? We could kill it and chop it up into small pieces, but as tempting as that sounds, there would be utter chaos, so that won't work. The alternative is to tame this ravenous beast; get it to stop killing people by getting rid of the evil caretakers who were abusing this poor animal.

Finally, we need to identify what is killing so many people unnecessarily, make the ones responsible take accountability by firing those who need to be fired, jailing those who need to be jailed and re-educate the remaining misguided souls who want to do a better job of taking care of us. We need to put the practice of medicine back into the hands of the doctors, give the nurses a lot more dignity and respect and partner up with the consumers in creating a team effort to focus on patient safety in hospitals and other nursing facilities. Once we make hospitals, clinics, nursing homes and doctors' offices into a safe haven for solving problems and maintaining good health, we can work toward ending wasteful spending and then begin providing a universal health insurance plan that guarantees coverage for every American citizen or legal resident.

How do we renovate a Burning House?

The Biblical accounting of the 26,000-mile long sea monster, lying at the bottom of all of the oceans wrapped around the entire planet illustrates the fact that there lurks a potentially destructive monster beneath the surface in all human endeavors. We usually sail along oblivious to what lurks beneath in the hidden depths until the monster raises its ugly head and capsizes the boat. Then we are in a middle of a crisis and the political leaders decide it's time for action.

So, how do we renovate a burning house? The answer is quite simple. First, we have to put out the fire. The health care "system" (if you really need to call it that) is fragmented, sloppy, bloated with high priced technology, overloaded with harmful drugs and profit driven by people who shamelessly engage in price gouging knowing how desperately people want to live. Pharmaceuticals are pushing feel good drugs for every conceivable symptom without any concern over side effects. The average person who is under medical care for chronic conditions is taking so many pills we have a new diagnosis on the books called "polypharmacy". This is a condition whereby the drug interactions cause loss of memory, loss of vitality, dizziness and mental confusion with urinary and fecal incontinence. When one examines the list of medications, one often finds that there are pills prescribed for the side effects of other pills, which the doctor prescribed for the side effects of other pills.

Aside from the big pharmaceutical companies assailing the public with billions of dollars' worth of overpriced harmful drugs (many costing $15 or more for each pill), hospitals, rehab facilities and nursing homes are causing bedsores, fractures, infections with gangrene, pulmonary embolism, choking, anemia, starvation, dehydration, traumatic brain hemorrhage, narcotic overdose, adverse drug reactions, burns, brain damaged babies and death from all sorts of treatable conditions. As mentioned previously these complications arise from incompetently performed procedures like sloppy technique, failure to provide basic nursing services, failure to monitor, failure to report changes in clinical condition, failure to respond to emergencies in a timely manner, giving the wrong medication or wrong dose, using equipment that is in disrepair, failure to train staff on proper operation of equipment, failure to maintain continuing education requirements of professional staff, operating on the wrong body part and leaving surgical products behind in the body.

Therefore, the Congress needs to hold hearings to learn about the common errors that are occurring in every hospital and nursing facility across the country. They then need to begin codifying basic standards of human decency, i.e. whereby it would be illegal to keep a patient waiting more than three minutes before answering a call bell. Thousands of people suffer severe injury and death because no one answered the patient's call for help and this happens in every hospital and nursing home. Therefore, unless the lawmakers wake up to these harsh realities, health care will just become more expensive and more destructive and once the Leviathan raises its head and swamps the boat there will be nothing left to reform.

Political Wind – the Baucus Banter

"**Research documenting poor quality of care received by patients in the U.S. is shocking.**"

No argument there; the situation is indeed shocking, but it should only be a big surprise to Rip Van Winkle, who fell asleep for forty years. Senator Baucus et al sound as though this was some sort of new revelation. However, the horrible quality of health care in American hospitals and nursing homes has been in the public eye for more than ten years. Hospital executives paid lip service to making changes and hired patient safety officers and the public and Congress remained silent; but the result was that the number of unnecessary deaths almost doubled. While it is possible that there was better reporting of fatal medical errors by the time Healthgrades released its report in 2004, it remains that the hospital executive quest for self-improvement was a colossal failure.

"**A 2003 Rand Corporation study found that adults received recommended care for many illnesses only 55 percent of the time. Needed care for diabetes was delivered only 45 percent of the time and for pneumonia only 39 percent of the time.**"

The results of the Rand Corporation study show us that HMO's have been successful in their bid to deny medical care to those who need it.

"Medicare and most other insurers continue to pay for more visits, tests, imaging services, and procedures, regardless of whether the treatment is effective or necessary, and pay even more when treatment results in subsequent injury or illness. Providers are not consistently encouraged to coordinate patients' care or to supply preventive and primary care services, even though such actions can improve quality of care and reduce costs. Rewarding providers that furnish better quality care, coordinate care, and use resources more judiciously could reduce costs and, most importantly, better meet the health care needs of millions more American patients."

The Senator did not present the entire picture. To begin with, the health care organizations are providing higher numbers of visits, tests and imaging selectively to those with fee-for-service with co-pay health plans. People with prepaid health maintenance plans receive less care because it is more profitable that way. Those who serve the Medicare and Medicaid population receive the smallest fees and must depend on high volume to reap desired profit levels. Thus, the visits tend to be shorter and rushed; so that many medical practitioners have no time for such services as taking a thorough history, conducting a careful physical examination and listening to the patient's complaints and concerns. Therefore, medical providers tend to overload the affluent population with unnecessary tests and treatments while they deprive the poor of quality services with a short shrift.

Finally, Senator Baucus and his colleagues do not seem to know how to define quality when it comes to health care. When they learn it they will be able to codify basic standards of care. Here are some questions that the Senate Committee on Health

Care Reform should ask when they conduct hearings with leaders of health care provider organizations:

<u>Clinics and Office Practices</u>
1. How much time on average does each doctor spend with each patient?
2. Do your patients see the same doctors on each visit for continuity?
3. How long do your patients have to wait on average to see the doctor for a specific appointment?
4. Do your patients have access to their doctors by telephone or email to ask questions?
5. Are your prescriptions block printed or typed for clarity?
6. Do you employ registered nurses for patient teaching and health counseling?
7. If you employ physician assistants or nurse practitioners, does the attending physician see the patient periodically or only when there is a severe problem?
8. Do you provide preventive health services like nutrition counseling and exercise programs?

<u>Hospitals and Nursing Facilities</u>
1. What is the average waiting time in your emergency room for a patient to see a doctor (hospitals only)?
2. How many unfilled registered nurse positions do you have?
3. What actions are you taking for registered nurse retention and recruitment?
4. Could you pass an accreditation inspection if they entered your building today?

5. Does your professional staff have all of their continuing education requirements up to date?
6. Do all patients have treatment plans and nursing care plans?
7. Do you have safe staffing levels on your floors and units at all times?
8. If you have an unsafe staffing situation do you notify the patients' families?
9. Do you have fall risk assessments on all patients?
10. Do have full implementation on all fall prevention protocols, including one-to-one sitters when indicated?
11. Do your registered nurses know their patients' conditions and what symptoms to look for?
12. Do your registered nurses know the drugs they are dispensing and what are the possible side effects and drug interactions?
13. Do you have bedsore risk assessments on all patients?
14. Do you have full implementation on all pressure ulcer prevention protocols with specialty mattresses, skin assessments every shift and turning and repositioning every two hours when indicated?
15. Do your attending doctors see their patients first before issuing orders upon admission?
16. How long do your patients have to wait on average for a nurse to answer their calls for help?
17. Do your nurses answer all calls for help within three minutes?

As of now, one of the most identifiable problems as a root cause of the deterioration in patient safety in hospitals and nursing facilities is the nursing shortage; and there are many other conditions leading to careless deadly mistakes. Senator Baucus and the rest of the Congress were supposed to stop the political whitewashing, begin to uncover the real problems and learn from real experts how to solve them. Congress needs to work toward setting standards of care rather than allowing the industry to police itself by consensus of like-minded professionals. The self-regulation system has been a dismal failure and has cost millions of lives. Therefore, Congress needs to form a special committee on health care guided by experts and consumers, find out what's really going on and start hammering out ways to stop the killing of 550 people daily. That is the equivalent of two commercial airliners falling out of the sky every day due to negligence and/or equipment failure.

The Baucus Vision Needed More Focus

According to the White Paper, there is a consensus among Americans about how to reform health care:
1. Every American should have health coverage with a mix of public and private health plans;
2. The government must institute policies that will slow the rate of growth in health spending over time;
3. The quality of care must improve, and payment systems should better aligned incentives to foster a focus on providing better care rather than more care;
4. Our system must also encourage wellness and the prevention of disease through early detection, modification of risk factors, and encouragement of healthy lifestyle choices;
5. When illness prevention fails, the focus should be on

care coordination;
6. Health reform includes the recognition that health care is a shared responsibility between government, employers and individuals.

First, I like the idea of health coverage for every American. However, the Senators and House Members needed to understand the difference between the insurance and health care industries. At one time, there was a clear delineation between insurance companies and health care providers. Blue Cross/Blue Shield was the largest insurer and the plan was simple. The insurance covered all medical costs while the patient stayed in the hospital and the people paid out of pocket for all outpatient visits. The insurers never told doctors how to practice medicine; they just paid the bills. Then everything spiraled out of control; doctors' fees went through the roof with the new age of specialization and technology explosion and insurance companies came forward with prepaid health maintenance plans and took over control of doctors and hospitals.

Initially, the idea seemed appealing. I recall listening to a presentation from a HIP sales rep in 1988. He said, "Your employer will pay a certain amount each month for health maintenance and we take care of everything you need with our doctors and hospitals." The truth is that to call it "health maintenance" was a lie. They never did anything to promote healthy living and screening for disease prevention or early diagnosis and treatment. Instead, they pressured their doctors to cut costs by reducing the number of referrals to specialists and denied approval for surgical procedures. Therefore, while I agree with universal coverage, we needed to take measures to release the strangle hold that the insurance companies have on health care delivery.

Second, Senator Baucus did not tell us how he intends to slow the rate of growth of health spending in America. However, one way to make a huge dent in the slowing down the growth in health care spending is to slow down the proliferation of new drugs with more side effects causing more damage to vital organs. The pharmaceutical companies are feverishly pushing new chemical compounds to treat every disease known to humans. They hand over millions of dollars in research grants to get the results they want for FDA approval.

Notwithstanding that, such research is worthless because the financial backers have a strong stake in showing that their product is the latest new medical miracle, the corrupt FDA officials give their approval and we get yet another drug with a new patent that's no better than any of the others. What's more, the pharmaceutical reps will then invite thousands of doctors to go to professional conferences on cruises or to some exotic resort and those physicians will begin prescribing the worthless poison en mass. Then, the new "miracle cure" will cause more illness and death with damage to vital organs in thousands of unsuspecting victims thereby increasing health spending mostly on more drugs to counteract the side effects of the drugs taken for the side effects of other drugs taken for the side effects of other drugs.

Therefore, if the FDA takes just one drug of each category off the market we will save billions of dollars and tens of thousands of lives. Better yet, if doctors stop prescribing Ritalin and other amphetamines to rob children of their natural energy to make them more controllable in schools, we will save millions of dollars and thousands of children can have a chance to grow strong and healthy instead of having to institutionalize them because of amphetamine brain damage. Those would be great ways to "slow down health spending."

Third, "Better care rather than more care" is someone's feeble attempt at generating a new catchphrase. In the real world, it is utterly meaningless because disease driven medical care always comes down to a decision whether or not to proceed with high tech diagnostic test and/or surgery or to be conservative and play the let's wait and see game. Either way there is a risk, so more does not necessarily mean better, but waiting too long could cause death from a treatable condition. Then again, better care actually means having the doctor take a personal interest in the patient, listen to his or her concerns go over the options and the risks of each and let the patient make an informed decision. Of course this higher quality of care would require more of the doctor's time, so in this case more care is better care. Furthermore, if Congress really wants to improve health care in America they will have to get the Hospitals to stop killing 200,000 people per year (548 per day, 23 per hour) with their sloppy technique, fiscal mismanagement and careless mistakes.

Fourth, encouraging wellness and prevention with behavior modification are good concepts, but I don't' know how Congress can legislate them unless they plan on putting a ban on pizza (perish the thought!). Perhaps they should impose a tax surcharge on certain fast foods, so that it would be cheaper to order a "McTofu" burger with special sauce on a whole-wheat sesame bun for starters. On the other hand, maybe education would work, so that we can refocus our health education classes in public high schools with lessons on healthy diets and exercise rather than just handing out condoms. We would certainly slow the spending on teenage pregnancy and venereal disease.

Fifth, "care coordination" is another stupid buzzword. The straight talk equivalent is, "When all else fails, rely on the gatekeeper to keep people away from specialists, high tech diagnostics and surgery." However, if this rhetoric has anything to do with avoiding duplication of tests, I am all for it.

A common scenario is that Mr. Jones goes to his primary care provider (that's family doctor in plain English) and they take blood, send it to the lab and report that some of the numbers are abnormal. The family doctor tells Mr. Jones that he needs to see a kidney specialist. He goes to the specialist and they start by drawing blood to repeat the exact same test, because they want to be sure. I have always thought that this was wasteful and stupid, especially when both doctors use the same laboratory. Therefore, certainly, there is much duplication, but care coordination is not the answer because the replication always happens after the referral to the specialist. Thus, we need new rules that will say to the specialist, "If you want to repeat the test because you don't trust the referring physician, fine; then you can pay for it."

Finally, I agree with the shared responsibility concept, but Senator Baucus forgot to include hospital owners and executives, nursing home owners and administrators, doctors and nurses. They are the ones who are collectively killing more than 200,000 people per year and injuring hundreds of thousands more though negligent acts and neglect. If the government refuses to make them accountable for this mayhem, then how will shared responsibility between government, employers and individuals help to improve health and quality of care? We need real action based on a real working knowledge of the current state of affairs in all health care provider environments. Political grandstanding and buzzword rhetoric just doesn't cut it anymore.

What the Congressional "Call to Action" is

not Telling us

Focusing attention on prevention and wellness is a wonderful thought. However, Senator Baucus, in his "Call to Action" is missing several important points.

"E. FOCUSING ON PREVENTION AND WELLNESS

Chronic diseases — such as stroke, heart disease, cancer, and diabetes — are the most prevalent and preventable of all health problems and also the most costly. Nearly half (45 percent) of Americans suffer from one or more chronic conditions and chronic disease accounts for 70 percent of all deaths (more than 1.7 million people). In addition, increased rates of obesity and chronic disease are the primary cause of disability and diminished quality of life."

To wit, the harmful impact, personally and economically, of chronic diseases is well known and certainly, prevention by altering unhealthy life styles would have been a worthy educational campaign. However, the immediate concern has been better management of chronic diseases, which has always been fragmented with poor or no follow-up. First, Senator Baucus and his writers needed to have a better understanding of the definition of chronic illness. For example, stroke is not a chronic disease per say; it is an event of rupture or blockage of a blood vessel in the brain that causes severe disability requiring long-term rehabilitation. On the other hand, high blood pressure is a chronic disease that leads to stroke and the process of keeping one's blood pressures under control will prevent such events in most cases.

Second, the term "heart disease" also needed further

clarification because there are many different types of heart problems, some of which are life-style related and some of which are hereditary. For example, we know that there is a link between excessive amounts of low-density lipoproteins found in the average American diet and coronary insufficiency (blockage of the coronary arteries leading to heart attacks). One serious problem we face today is that pharmaceutical companies who market statins, with the approval of corrupt FDA officials, are trying to convince us that we all need to take statins to prevent heart attacks and strokes. Statins are a group of drugs like Crestor that reduce the amount of cholesterol in the blood and have known side effects causing muscle weakness, kidney damage and liver failure. Therefore, if we have an unchecked corrupt government bureaucracy that will allow the Statin makers to recommend that doctors prescribe such drugs indiscriminately based on one manufacturer-financed study, then how will Congress be able to affect any reforms? Hence government is part of the problem.

Third, cancer prevention is something that our body of knowledge in health care is ill equipped to handle. Most of the ideas are purely theoretical. We have some notions that stress management, diet and smoking cessation are contributing factors to prevention, but there are also environmental pollutants and hereditary factors over which we have no control. However, the most effective tools that we have in fighting this dreaded disease is early detection through periodic screening exams. We also need to take a serious look at the chemical ingredients in our foods, the pesticides on domestic produce and foreign imports, carcinogens like chlorine in our water supplies and high voltage electromagnetic fields, to name a few.

Fourth, I am not sure that diabetes is actually preventable

because it is purely genetic. In any case there are two basic types: juvenile onset and adult onset. The former has no prevention and the young patients must rely on meticulous management to avoid complications. The latter is also not preventable per say, but we can forestall its onset with diet and exercise. In other words, we each have a certain amount of insulin production over a lifetime. The more carbohydrates we consume the faster we use up our insulin supply. Once it is depleted, we become diabetic. The amount of insulin we can produce over time is hereditary, so different people run out of it at different ages and some die at a ripe old age before that problem occurs.

To sum up, prevention and wellness are issues that go beyond health care and if the government were to focus on it properly, there has to be reforms in environmental protection, education, commercial food preparation and FDA drug approval criteria. Government has to stop being part of the problem with its corrupt special interest-favoring policies and, in addition, get the hospitals and nursing facilities to stop killing so many people.

Quality Improvement: The Road to Nowhere

The "Call to Action" health care reform plan that Senator Baucus initiated in 2009 is replete with a single theme; using financial incentives to improve quality of care. Although it is still not clear how the Democratic Senator from Montana measured quality, he suggested that minimizing duplication of services, and diagnostic tests was the key. While eliminating wasteful spending would certainly have been helpful, focusing on this aspect alone belied the reason why we all agreed that American health care quality is in the toilet. Therefore, to improve the quality of care in America, we first have to get hospitals to stop the systematic massacre. It's not that hospital personnel are looking to kill anyone, but we keep having the same mistakes and accidents happening repeatedly in every hospital across America. What does that tell us? It tells us, as I have stated repeatedly, that there are a number of flaws in the design in both the architecture and methodology.

Furthermore, we are not dealing with rocket science or some abstract dilemma. Changing the method of paying physicians, setting up stricter controls by a primary care provider (PCP) or having "physician offices, inpatient hospitals, post-acute care settings, and others to collaborate and provide patient-centered care in a way that improves quality and saves money" is not going to do anything to eliminate all of the unnecessary and tragic carnage that has been taking place every year for several decades. The task is difficult, but once we eliminate all of the political buffoonery, we can see that it's very simple. We already know what's killing so many people in hospitals and nursing facilities; a long list of complications arising out of neglect, incompetence, fiscal irresponsibility and wanton disregard of patient safety.

There are many specific reasons for such occurrences, but overall, we have major flaws in how the corporate culture in America runs the day-to-day operations in hospitals and nursing homes. Hence, the root cause for all of the above is the management policies of each institution. For example, the greatest negative impact on hospital services is the nurse-to-patient ratio, fiscal management and professionals with too much autonomy and zero accountability.

Consequently, hospital and nursing facility management as a whole is a dismal failure, so if there are to be any meaningful reforms, Congress needs to start with this group of individuals and make them accountable for the unintended consequences of any professional misbehavior. We need for members of Congress and President Obama to understand and face what we are really dealing with in terms of the cost in human lives and suffering. Health Care Quality means providing necessary services in a competent timely manner with adequate supplies and technological equipment in good working order. Unless and until Congress codifies the standards that we need to ensure patient safety, all of the past hoopla about health care reform call to action will continue to be a long hard road to nowhere.

Wrap Up

The "first do no harm principle" of medical practice is still very much in the conversation of today's physicians. It starts with the Hippocratic Oath, still being said at every medical school graduation ceremony and remains as the daily mantra. However, it doesn't happen that way in reality. The intention is to do no harm with treatment, but when the doctor has nothing more to offer than, "Let's try this and see if it works;" with possible side effects ranging from diarrhea to liver and kidney damage and sudden death. Therefore, the credo is more like "take a shot in the dark and hope for the best."

Yet, there is still a lot that health care providers can do to make their services safer. It starts with assessing the patient's ability to negotiate the environment and take necessary precautions. Providers then have to make certain that there are no hazards like spills or frayed wires and that all equipment is in good working order. Moreover, the nurses have to respond immediately to calls for assistance. Additionally, the operating room staff have to stay on guard to avoid the surgical foul-ups and be extra careful when moving people around after surgery. People working in institutional settings too often lose sight of the fact that they are working in an environment that is inherently harmful to the people they serve. Every nurse, doctor, therapist and technician in every hospital and nursing facility has to go to work every day thinking that there are accidents waiting to happen. Then there might be less harm and more healing.

8. Reinventing the Reinvented Wheel

The Primary Care Folly

The first stated goal in the Baucus plan for reforming the "health care delivery system" was to "strengthen the role of primary care". However, the good senator seemed oblivious to the fact that the primary care concept had been around for about thirty years and had become an abject failure. The designation came about with the rise of the failed experiment called "managed care." Hence, the Managed Care Organizations (MCO) created the "primary care provider" (PCP) to act as gatekeeper to block access to specialists and hi tech diagnostic tests. This structure exists today as the main model for medical care delivery. The method of paying physicians varies from one MCO to another, but the PCP generally has a financial incentive for not making specialist referrals.

Consequently, the gatekeeper system has done little or nothing to improve the quality of health care. On the other hand, the gatekeepers do prevent many unnecessary procedures. The problem is that PCP's don't always make decisions based on what is best for the patient, and the question of whether more extensive and expensive treatment is necessary cannot be answered until the patient goes for the additional tests and receives the result. Therefore, one cannot know the consequence of not seeing a specialist for more definitive diagnostic investigation of the problem until either the symptoms subside or the patient becomes critically ill.

Accordingly, it is not clear what Senator Baucus and team were alluding to when they wrote about "**Strengthening the role of primary care. . .**" How do you strengthen a failed methodology? The logical step was to say, "We have tried it for more than three decades and the results were disastrous; so now it's time to try something totally different rather than a new variation of the same theme in order to keep the stakeholders' financial interests intact." Hence, the Senator wanted to shift the financial incentive to pay rewards for a favorable patient outcome. Without even getting into the ramifications of how we were going to define outcome and what we were going to measure it against to determine whether it was more or less favorable, this idea was really just reverting to the way doctors practiced medicine before the MCO's gummed up the works. The PCP got paid for the initial visit and referred the patient to a specialist for a definitive diagnosis, recommendations and initial treatment for the specific problem. Then the patient went back to the PCP for ongoing long-term management.

Moreover, the Senator's new catchphrase, "We need better care rather than more care. . ." is an oxymoron, because you cannot improve patient outcomes without access to available technology and specialty skills. For example, if you have ten patients who complain of severe headache and one of them has an operable cerebral aneurysm (a defective artery in the brain that is about to burst) you may have to scan all ten people in order to find the one who will die without immediate brain surgery. The other nine all had migraines and all of the expensive testing, of course, was negative. Although, the Senator expects the PCP to have the skills to correctly weed out the patient with suspected aneurysm, send him to a neurosurgeon and avoid unnecessary specialty services and testing on the other nine, sometimes it will happen that way and sometimes it won't. However, the PCP has to ask himself, "What if I'm missing something?" Thus, he ends up sending all ten patients to a neurologist who orders CAT scans on all of them. The bottom line is if you tell the PCP, "We will pay you extra for better outcomes," how will that change anything or reduce cost? The primary doctor will want to cash in on testing everybody to make sure he doesn't miss anything.

On the other hand, if you go to a PCP, who has a population of ten thousand members under his/her charge, and say, "We will pay you extra if you keep them healthier," You are making the assumption that a PCP and staff can engage in effective behavior modification of thousands of people. In theory, it sounds good, but in practice I don't know if the financial incentive is going to be enough to achieve this clinical transformation. The real motivation has to be the desire on the part of physicians based on compassion rather than greed or need. The Democrats don't seem to think that such a doctor exists. However, since every young doctor starts his/her career with a debt of about half a million dollars and has a desperate need to pay it off, perhaps the Senator should look at ways of providing reciprocal medical education debt forgiveness as an incentive for better outcomes.

Another problem is the availability of primary care providers. As of now, the medical profession is top heavy with specialists and suffers from severe shortages of family practitioners.

Finally, there are some health problems that actually make going to the PCP for a referral a waste of time and money. If a person wakes up in the morning with an eye infection from a contact lens, then it makes sense to go directly to the ophthalmologist and then notify the PCP. There has to be some flexibility to be effective in reducing duplication. Another example is gynecology and obstetrics; there is no reason why women should have to get a referral for such care. Thus, there are situations in which the need for a specialist is obvious, so there is a call for flexibility.

Briefly, no one can refute the ultimate goal of preventing the preventable diseases and providing specialty care and hi tech services only to those who need it. However, we don't live in a perfect world and frankly, I would be happy if we can get through the next hour without doctors and nurses killing someone by mistake. However, if we are to analyze the problem accurately we need to see that heath care delivery is a big chaotic profit-driven mess and we need to clean it up by first getting rid of horses who drop their manure as they walk rather than to continue walking behind them with a shovel. Therefore, there is one simple solution to start a real reform: get the insurance companies out of medical practice.

The Patient Centered Medical Home: The Same Wolves in Sheep's Clothing

Shortly after the 2008 presidential election, Aetna and Partners-in-Care jointly announced a "new" health care model called the "Patient-Centered Medical Home (PCMH)". The press release stated, "**. . . the model emphasized the role of the primary care physician (PCP) in managing and coordinating patient care across a range of care providers, including specialists and hospitals.**"[20] Maybe I am missing something here, but this is exactly how the HMO's had set up medical care almost Fifty years ago; the primary care physician (PCP), also called the "gatekeeper" decided what specialists and other services to recommend. The trick to lowering health care

---

[20] http://www.marketwatch.com

costs was to pay a per capita rate to the PCP whether he saw the member or not and charge him back for every referral to a specialist or subscription for durable medical equipment and supplies. Therefore, the physician would make more money for providing less care. This was a scheme to provide financial incentives to cause doctors to deny entitled access to health care under the guise of discouraging unnecessary tests and specialty visits. The result was pandemic deviations from the professional standards of care.

Moreover, the timing of this so-called new model, PCMH, is interesting. Since Obama's election victory, there was a brand new media frenzy called "Health Care Reform". The public was now focusing on everything about the health care industry that they despised; especially HMO's. During the campaign, Obama talked about how an HMO denied his mother vital medical care and contributed to her health deterioration. Therefore, it was likely that the people at Aetna, PIC, Humana and others were worried. Hence, Aetna was going to pay extra money to the PCP for additional time spent in tracking the specialty care to see if the patient was following any new recommendations and avoid duplication of services. However, this sounded like more of the same except for the part about punishing the PCP for making the referral to the specialist or prescribing medical equipment.

The press release provided us with three-bulleted descriptions of how this "new" approach would work.
2. "Implement a Medical Home model which places the patient's personal physician in charge of all the patient's care needs, including arranging and tracking care with other qualified professionals at all stages including acute care, chronic care, preventive services and even end of life care

services;

3. "Use the PIC-developed 'Physician-Guided Care Coordination' approach to care. Aetna would reimburse the PCP for taking time to make sure that all of the patient's caregivers are aware of and following the treatment plan prescribed by that PCP;
4. "Provide physicians with detailed clinical data provided by Aetna Health Analytics and through its subsidiary Active Health Management, to identify changes that may be needed and to help assure that the patients receive the right care at the right time and place."

The first description doesn't offer anything new. This is exactly the definition of the PCP that existed since the 1970's.

The second bullet defines the PCP as the person in charge of the care plan and has the final say regarding any specialist recommendations. It seemed as if elective diagnostic tests and surgery still required prior approval for full coverage and this blurb merely told the PCP to fulfill his or her obligation, which has been the same for more than three decades.

The third "innovation" sounded like the same physician practice profiling that has been around since the year of the flood. Moreover, making sure that the patients receive the right care at the right time and place really means, "We are still going to try to get away with denying care whenever possible."

Finally, there is not one word mentioned in the Aetna-PIC press release about holistic approaches or allowing the patient to have any say or participation in formulating the care plan. It is the same autocratic "blindly follow doctor's orders or we won't pay" crap that the HMO's have been shoving down our throats for decades. Oh, but now they are calling it a "medical home" instead of the provider's office. It's as if they are telling us, "Come to mommy and daddy, tell us your troubles and we'll make it all go away." Well, if I decided to move into my new medical home, would I at least get to pick the curtains?

The Spin Doctor's Paradise

The definition of PCMH that the C.E.O. of Med Net One proffered on a Comcast video is that it is a new model of health care whereby physicians re-focus themselves on the patient. It sounds like these HMO executives are congratulating themselves for being so magnanimous as to encourage their physicians to provide some real customer service. Thus, this so-called "medical home" movement is nothing more than reverting by rhetoric back to the time when physician care was the family doctor, general practitioner Marcus Welby type. He worked out of his home and took a loving interest in all of his patients. When they came to see him, they were like guests in the doctor's home. It all started with Hippocrates saying some 3,000 years ago, "First, do no harm." Thus, this new bogus advertising gimmick proves what King Solomon, the wisest human that ever lived, once said; "There is nothing new under the sun."

It's interesting to note that during and prior to the 1950's, most physicians in smaller communities conducted their practices in their homes. Most people could afford the price of a visit because physicians were charging what people could afford. However, then came the greedy HMO's, under the guise of decreasing the cost of health care without decreasing quality, who wedged themselves in between us and our doctors and took over everything. They were very successful, in decreasing cost when it came to paying the physicians and hospitals, but they also succeeded in charging us more. So now, we pay 250% more for health care while doctors are making less money per visit than they did thirty years ago. Ironically, this trend actually started with single payer government health insurance for the poor and elderly; Medicaid and Medicare, which paved the way for the prepaid health plans. Physicians, not wanting to give up control of their professional lives to corporate greed, themselves formed incorporated physician groups. At first, they did it to protect the patient from non-professionals interfering with medical orders, but alas, they too became mostly profit-driven and joined the corporate culture.

Hence, we now have the so-called "medical home" where we can expect to see "Marcus Welby, M.D." greeting us as we step over the threshold into yesteryear. Of course, now there is a new upgrade in the programming, such as electronic patient files, a nutritionist for those special diets, a nurse-consultant, a mental health counselor for stress management and life style modification, and maybe even a personal trainer thrown in for special exercise programs along with various medical specialists. This all sounds wonderful, but the only thing new about it is the name; back in the 1970's they called it holistic health care. Multi-specialty groups have also been around for decades, so what is new about PCMH? The answer is nothing but the catch phrase. What is mind boggling about all this is that they seriously expected the "we need health reform now" Obama-bots to buy into this medical swindle as part of the health reform plan. I suppose the HMO executives needed to make us believe that they have become part of the new solution or that they even cared about health.

Moreover, the advocates of "medical home" say that the family practitioners are going to get more pay for providing all of this extra stuff, but who is going to pay the check for the meal with all the frills? One family practitioner in the Bronx, New

York said that certain HMO's approached him and wanted an investment of $30,000 to create a "medical home" for a fourteen dollar per visit increase in the reimbursement. Thus, it looked like these medical robber barons wanted to stick it to our doctors and their patients once again by asking them to eat the cost of renovations for re-packaging the same old shoe, while they intended to gouge the taxpayers to cough up the extra money for this new "health care reform".

In short, the principle of change through insanity is, "If at first you don't succeed, just repeat the same failure with a new spin. Thus, what should we do when a failing industry has a middleman that exploits the suppliers and gouges the customers? Get rid of him. Without this middleman, there would no longer be anyone running interference between the doctor and patient. On the other hand we also need physicians to conform to patient safety standards with elimination of duplicative diagnostic studies and unnecessary procedures.

The process of Change has to Change

After the election of President Obama, the health care reform activity fast turned into a special interest feeding frenzy. As the previous administration ended, the lobbyists were scurrying about in the political sewers of Washington, D.C. getting ready to bring their clients' visions of health care reform to the attention of lawmakers. The insurance companies wanted to make certain that they could still sell their health plans at a profit within the proposed universal coverage system; the pharmaceuticals wanted to continue to sell their toxic drugs and bring more to market and the hospital and physician groups wanted relief from malpractice lawsuits without disturbing the status quo of self-regulation. If you had lifted up the big rock, you would have seen the vermin scurrying about on Capitol Hill wining and dining our elected officials to push for a health care reform package that would inure to the benefit of those who made the largest soft campaign contributions. So we have seen that this new push for better health care in America has been the same old D.C. politics as usual.

To continue, there were four major interest groups reported in the news media that were lining up at the trough: 1) insurance companies; 2) pharmaceutical firms; 3) physicians and hospitals; 4) Consumer advocacy groups. First, the insurance companies were interested in universal coverage through an insurance exchange as proposed in the Baucus plan if purchase of a health plan became mandatory for every American. This way they could spread their risks over a large population. The whole idea from an actuarial perspective is to cover a young, healthy population so that their premiums would pay for care of the sick with a few million left over at the end of each year. The insurance carriers also argued that the premiums and deductibles would remain in check by competition in a free market, and that they should continue to be allowed to own and/or control medical practice and hospital systems. In other words, if it was going to be business as usual with more healthy customers mandated by the new laws, they were all for it; and we knew from Hillary's past colossal failure that passage of a new health reform act had no chance if the insurance companies opposed it. Of course, they wanted to reduce costs, but outcomes were not part of their equation.

Second, the big pharmas had their own agenda; they wanted to continue selling their drugs. They also want to continue spending millions and reaping billions bringing us more new drugs; with improved efficacy and higher toxicity. If you have noticed any of the drug commercials on Television lately you have heard lines spoken by some actor pretending to be a patient saying, "I had such a difficult time with my breathing and energy level until I started taking 'Toxicity Plus'. Now I can breathe easier and I have the energy to play with my grandchildren." Then the next scene shows a middle-aged man or woman pushing a kid on a swing followed by a rapid-fire list of potential side effects coming from the narrator saying, "People with heart, kidney or liver problems should not take Toxicity Plus as irreversible heart, kidney and liver damage have been known to occur. Pregnant and nursing mothers should not take Toxicity Plus." Then the actor comes back smiling and says, "Toxicity Plus has given me a new lease on life, and it can do the same for you. Ask your doctor if Toxicity Plus is right for you." Then, of course, the doctor that you are supposed to consult has just returned from an all-expense paid Caribbean cruise, courtesy of the makers of "Toxicity Plus" and he has a package of starter pills to give you for free, just because he's a nice guy.

Third, physicians and hospitals have a huge stake in the status quo regarding self-regulation. Certainly, no one in the health care provider industry wants to cause death and disabling injury. However, in the trenches it is impossible to see the big picture, so in the normal course of business, people fall out of bed, develop bedsores, receive the wrong medication, undergo someone else's surgical procedure, walk around with sponges and instruments left behind, and suffer from a long list of other mistakes and mishaps. On the other hand, if any one were to suggest that government pass laws mandating basic standards of care, the outcry from physicians and hospital management would be deafening. "You can't legislate standards of care!" they would argue because medicine is an art and not a science. Meanwhile, hospital policy, physician behavior and individual nursing errors cause all of the mayhem. Thus, self-regulation has failed and the health care system is the fifth leading cause of death in America today. Therefore we need legislation that will codify the standards of care and hold people as well as corporations accountable for violations.

Finally, the consumer advocacy groups say they want patient safety and universal coverage to be the top priorities, but are they really speaking up for all of us consumers? For example, there is an advertisement aired on TV touting United Health as the best provider for Medicare supplemental insurance citing AARP endorsement and saying, "This is the only health plan endorsed by the AARP, an organization that you trust." This situation begs the question, "How can a consumer advocacy group have any credibility if it is making money with endorsements from the companies that they are supposed to be watching?" The bottom line is that consumer advocacy is a silent voice in health care because we have not seen any activity to counteract the media blitz coming from the other special interests.

To sum up, we can see where this whole push for health care reform is going; nowhere. The reason is that the agent of change is the same political process; campaign promises, followed by a call to action, followed by meetings with professional lobbyists representing all of the special interests. The result will be more of the same poor quality with possibly some resolution regarding insurance coverage and premiums being more competitive. The only way that we can have any meaningful transformation is to change the process of change.

Health Care Reform Needs Reform: The

Obama House Party

According to the New York Times[21], in 2008, shortly after the election, President Obama asked a dozen of his former campaign volunteers to get together at a house party and discuss what's wrong with the health care system. They all said interesting things and gave what seemed like heartfelt opinions. However, not one of them touched on the heart of the problem in health care regarding the number of unnecessary deaths per year. Moreover, these members of the new Obama nation seemed oblivious to the fact that simply being admitted to a hospital incurred a 1 in 500 risk of death.

This impromptu consumer think tank said that they hate insurance companies (no big surprise there). They complained about coverage exclusions and maternity benefits that required a six-month waiting period before conception. They also agreed that health care is a right and that the profit motive is impeding access to quality care. There was also a comment about the lack of coverage for screening and preventive medicine and about the need for internet based health record informatics within a secured network.

Although the group identified some valid concerns, this informal gathering was a waste of time, if this was supposed to provide any useful input. Obama's first knee-jerk reaction should have been, "Tell me something I don't know." Obama and his followers have either been unbelievably naïve or living in denial like 200 million of their fellow Americans because there was not one single word about medical and nursing negligence in hospitals, nursing homes and other health care facilities and

---

[21] http://www.nytimes.com/2008/12/23/health/23health.html?_r=2

organizations. This bizarre phenomenon never ceases to boggle my mind. When considering the number of people adversely affected by medical and nursing mistakes we can ascertain the 84% of Americans have fallen victim to health care error or know someone who has. Perhaps this group of twelve belong to the other 16% comprised exclusively of clueless Kool-Aid drinkers.

In conclusion, the president and congress still need to consult with experts on patient safety and prevention of medical errors, and since Obama said that he wanted to hear people's stories, he should listen to doctors, nurses and the victims of their mistakes. He would soon discover (if he doesn't already know) that the entire system of self-regulation is a deadly failure.

Doesn't Anybody Want to Prevent Medical Errors?

Once the new congress and President were in full swing, it was clear that health care reform was not the first priority since they did the stimulus package first. Apparently, all of the new and not-so-new leaders seemed oblivious to the continued carnage taking place in America's hospitals vis-à-vis the never-ending never events. After a flurry of political activity and mass media frenzy people continued to die at the rate of 23 per hour. So why doesn't the public express its outrage? The simple answer is that there is no drama as there is with a plane crash, train wreck or a terrorist bombing. It's just statistics; like hearing about the number of people who die on America's highways. The public accepts it as casualties of our modern way of life. However, the big difference is that traffic issues are constantly under review with law enforcement vigorously pursuing traffic violators, so we can say that government is doing all that it can to minimize traffic mishaps. However, we don't have that same diligence for patient safety even though deaths due to hospital mistakes far outnumber those on the highways. The hospital industry remains "self-regulated" in spite of its colossal failures.

Moreover, we can see from the news media the total lackluster response to the revelations made about hospital and medical errors in the United States. There was an editorial in the Post Bulletin of Minnesota by Bill Boynton[22] that says, "The Minnesota Adverse Health Care Reporting Act was passed in 2003 on the recommendation of the state's hospital and nurse associations. The legislation was proposed after the Institute of Medicine reported that up to 98,000 Americans were dying each year from preventable medical errors." What the author failed to mention was that the IOM reported the 98,000 death rate in 1999.

The fact that it took four years for the Minnesota lawmakers to pass legislation mandating the disclosure of hospital/medical/nursing errors is mind boggling. Furthermore, notwithstanding the claim that public disclosure of health care negligence is causing providers to be more careful, the reporting was after the fact and did not address the massive deviations from appropriate standards of care. Although Mr. Boynton seemed ready to slap all of the major players in Minnesota on the back with a hearty "well done", we need to wait until we see some hard data before we get too happy with mandated disclosure, especially if that is the only legislative measure in place for improving patient safety.

---

[22]
http://www.postbulletin.com/newsmanager/templates/localnews_story.asp?z=12&a=382406

In summary, I am a voice in the wilderness crying out for mandated patient safety standards as the first priority in achieving real health care reform. Why should people have to continue to risk wrongful death by going into a hospital or doctor's office for treatment?

The Reality Check

"Tens of millions of Americans are uninsured because of rising costs. Over 45 million Americans—including over 8 million children—lack health insurance. Eighty percent of the uninsured are in working families. Even those with health coverage are struggling to cope with soaring medical costs. Skyrocketing health care costs are making it increasingly difficult for employers, particularly small businesses, to provide health insurance to their employees."

The above paragraph from one of Obama's campaign speeches didn't tell us what was really going on with regard to the plight of the uninsured. People without coverage usually use the emergency room as the family doctor for all medical problems. Federal law requires that no patient can be turned away for lack of insurance or money and hospitals have to eat the cost of providing care. Furthermore, municipal hospitals run by state, county and city governments must accept their own admissions as well as all of those being transferred from the private sector. Add to this crowd the twenty million illegal aliens who are entitled to health care under the same laws, and we have about 65 million uninsured people residing in the United States.

Additionally, Part of the reason why we have skyrocketing health care costs is the fact that the uninsured will get emergency room treatment for a common cold for a total charge of $600. The cost for the same treatment in a private clinic or doctor's office is about $60. Moreover, there is another federal law, the Hill-Burton Act, which requires the U.S. Treasury to cover the shortfall of any hospital that is unable to collect for treating uninsured, non-paying patients. Hence there is a financial incentive for hospitals to register every minor complaint as an emergency, so most hospitals now have in-house walk-in clinics staffed by E.R. doctors and nurses and charge emergency room rates.

Therefore, we need only one government to immediately reduce the cost of health treatment for common ailments; provide coverage that requires appropriate lower-cost treatment for non-emergent ailments. The uninsured are currently receiving hospital based care for all medical problems and the government is paying for it already at a much higher cost as mentioned above. Once we get these folks into a health plan to shift them away from utilizing the emergency room as the family doctor, the government will save billions of dollars every year because they will have reduced the cost per emergency encounter from $600 to $60.

Moreover, we do not need a whole new system of reimbursement. All we need is to remove the maximum income exclusion for Medicaid and charge premiums on a sliding scale according to income. The important point here is that health providers should no longer be receiving emergency rates for non-emergency treatment. This would result in a 90% reduction in the cost of primary care for the 45 million plus uninsured folks in the United States.

Second, there is the cost of providing free medical care to illegal aliens that has been bankrupting all of the Southwestern states and municipalities as well as the federal government. We have not heard anything from the current administration about the cost of providing non-emergent emergency health care to illegal aliens, none of whom have ever had to undergo go any kind of health screening prior to entry. Notwithstanding the insanity of giving such entitlements to people who disregard our laws and add a myriad of social problems, we face the same dilemma of paying 1,000% more in emergency rooms for minor injuries and ailments that could easily be treated in doctors' offices. Thus, if our government officials lack the courage to enforce our laws then they can at least re-direct those who don't need emergency care into clinics and save billions of dollars per year.

In conclusion, the approximately 65 million people who are uninsured in this country are currently receiving health care mostly through emergency rooms and all levels of government are already paying the cost at ten times what it cost to treat the insured. Therefore we don't need the Obama-Biden spending machine to re-invent the wheel. We can immediately start spending 90% less money by giving every uninsured person a Medicaid card and charge for it on a sliding scale according to income.

The Reinvented Wheel: Obama's Health Reform Law

To be certain, health care in America needed a lot of reform in the way that providers conduct themselves and operate their facilities. We also need to cover the uninsured so the taxpayers can stop paying for emergency room usage for what should be office visits. However, the political health reform plan as passed into law in 2010 and upheld by the United States Supreme Court in 2012 is full of fancy rhetoric with no substance. The lack of accomplishment is no big surprise because politicians usually talk a lot, say little and do even less. The truth is that we don't need the U.S. government to wipe our noses. We have an infrastructure. What needed was for congress to pass laws setting standards of decency based on input from professionals in patient safety and making health care decision makers personally accountable for the lives they destroy. Hence, to say that the government is going to bring about improvement in outcomes with information technology, better disease management and the like is a scam because the politicians have never had any clue about the disease process and the health care system. Therefore, we shall take a closer look at the claims of creating a new health care utopio.

"Invest in electronic health information technology systems."

Undoubtedly, electronic paperless record keeping is the wave of the present and future in all industries and there are some aspects about health informatics that enhance patient safety, like computerized prescriptions. On the other hand we need to make certain that the patient doesn't get robbed of the ability to look for the best price for medications. I have often taken my written prescription to two or more different drug stores and saved hundreds of dollars by comparative shopping. Thus, any electronic prescribing system should tell the consumer where to get the best price for the medicine.

On the other hand, electronic record keeping may save provider time, but computer charting systems are not uniform and are often confusing. There is a huge learning curve for inputting data and input errors are rampant. After having seen numerous printouts from a variety of systems, I can tell you that it is often easier to read hand written notes. There are also a lot of boiler plate notes that nurses and doctors use so that progress records are often meaningless. Therefore, if there is going to be a substantial increase in computerized charting there must be some minimum standards required such as:

1. Progress notes must be uniquely typed for each patient—there has to be a thought process behind the words with regard to a particular patient's condition and clinical changes;
2. Printouts must be in narrative from that simply replaces hand written words with type;
3. If any lab work or other diagnostic test is pending, the computer will continue to prompt the user to view the results;
4. The computer will prompt the user for any medications that are due and not given;
5. The computer will prompt the user for vital sign checks and any periodic observations required by order or standards of care;
6. The computer will prompt the user for any actions required by any of the nursing care plans, such as turning the patient from side to side to prevent bed sores.

Thus, we can see that the health informatics industry needs to rise to the occasion to program reminders for interventions required by the standards of care. This will force nurses, doctors and other allied professionals to focus on the duty owed to the patient at all times.

"Support disease management programs. Over seventy-five percent of total health care dollars are spent on patients with one or more chronic conditions, such as

diabetes, heart disease, and high blood pressure. Many patients with chronic diseases benefit greatly from disease management programs, which help patients manage their condition and get the care they need. Barack Obama and Joe Biden will require that plans that participate in the new public plan, Medicare or the Federal Employee Health Benefits Program (FEHBP) utilize proven disease management programs. This will improve quality of care and lower costs, as well."

This paragraph begs the question, "What is a disease management program?" In other words, what did Obama want to do that was different from what was already being done for people who belonged to a paid health plan? If someone had diabetes, for example, he would receive medication to lower his blood sugar, be given a special diet to follow, a regimen of daily exercise, obtain a test device to monitor the blood glucose and visit the doctor for follow up visits once every month. Keeping the blood sugar under control would avoid most complications of the disease and reduce co morbidity. However, the result has always been up to the patient. He/she has to comply with the daily regimen; if not, the disease management will fail. Success depends entirely upon the patient's ability to sacrifice immediate desire for long term benefits. I knew a doctor once who would say to his non-compliant patients, "If you don't care about your health, why should I?" Therefore, if President Obama wants the federal government to intercede in the area of individual behavior modification for better outcomes, federal law enforcement agents would have to have a new mandate.

"Coordinate and integrate care. Rates of chronic diseases have skyrocketed in the last 2 decades. Over 133 million Americans have at least one chronic disease. With proper care, the onset and progression of these diseases can be contained for many years. In addition to the needless suffering and early death they cause, these chronic conditions cost a staggering $1.7 trillion yearly. Barack Obama and Joe Biden will support providers to put in place care management programs and encourage team care through implementation of medical home type models that will improve coordination and integration of care of those with chronic conditions."

This paragraph was pact with fancy rhetoric, but with no substance. It was like a breath of hot air. Coordinating and integrating care is having a primary care gatekeeper to make decisions about specialist referrals. The reference to improving coordination and integration of care of those with chronic conditions sounds like another way of saying "disease management programs." This is a reinvention of the reinvented wheel. If Obama really wanted to improve disease management, he should have emphasized the idea of personal responsibility and accountability and encourage the formation of more support groups where people with chronic diseases can help each other, like "Diabetics Anonymous". The new political rhetoric vis-à-vis health care was beginning to sound too much like "Big Brother is watching you".

Wrap Up

The idea of primary care started more than a century ago when doctors could do little more than assist a mother with the birth of a child; remove a gangrenous limb to save a life and help someone die with less pain and more dignity. This was the role of the family doctor, who took an interest in people and went to their homes in the middle of the night to break a fever, ease some pain and make a decision about whether there was a need to go to the hospital.

Today, in the second decade of the new millennium, we have greater technology, but the same ailments and complaints. People live about thirty years longer on average, but the cost of longer life for an aging population is about to bankrupt our society. Thus the people in control of health care policy decided to go back to the "doctor knows best" Marcus Welby, M.D. approach to roll back the clock and the cost of care. There is also an emphasis on "primary care" to encourage family practitioners, internists and pediatricians to treat most ailments without referring to specialists. Of course, people would still go to specialists when there is an obvious need for surgical intervention or when symptoms persist and the primary doctor can't figure it out, but the PCP's now have the incentive to avoid utilizing higher cost health care.

Hence, when a patient's blood pressure is suddenly too high, the PCP will usually prescribe medication to lower it without trying to determine the root cause. The process of arriving at the correct therapeutic dosages without causing more damage with side-effects is more trial-and-error than anything else. So, in many cases, the treatment causes more harm than good.

In conclusion, the task of government now is to effectively block seniors from having access to high technology diagnostics and treatment and sell this package of earlier death to the general public in a way that will make us believe that we are getting higher quality at less cost. Consequently, we are seeing phony rhetorical buzz terms like "patient centered medical homes" to improve "coordination and integration." If the politicians were to tell us that medical care has become overpriced, sloppy and dangerous, then we could relate to measures that would correct these systemic deficiencies, like patient safety standards. However, no one wants to make the health industry accountable, so they must pretend that they are inventing some new way to make it more efficient and affordable.

9. From Lip to Law

The Whitehouse Wisdom

As the Patient Protection and Affordable Care Bill was being drafted, the Obama machine cranked up its internet campaign for public support. The following is an email from Obama and my response.

The White House, Washington
Good afternoon,

You are receiving this email because you signed up at WhiteHouse.gov. My staff and I plan to use these messages as a way to directly communicate about important issues and opportunities, and today I have some encouraging updates about health care reform.

The Vice President and I just met with leaders from the House of Representatives and received their commitment to pass a comprehensive health care reform bill by July 31.

We also have an unprecedented commitment from health care industry leaders, many of whom opposed health reform in the past. Monday, I met with some of these health care stakeholders, and they pledged to do their part to reduce the health care spending growth rate, saving more than two trillion dollars over the next ten years -- around $2,500 for each American family. Then on Tuesday, leaders from some of America's top companies came to the White House to showcase innovative ways to reduce health care costs by improving the health of their workers.

Now the House and Senate are beginning a critical debate that will determine the health of our nation's economy and its families. This process should be transparent and inclusive and its product must drive down costs, assure quality and affordable health care for everyone, and guarantee all of us a choice of doctors and plans.

Reforming health care should also involve you. Think of other people who may want to stay up to date on health care reform and other national issues and tell them to join us here:

http://www.whitehouse.gov/EmailUpdates

Health care reform can't come soon enough. We spend more on health care than any country, but families continue to struggle with skyrocketing premiums and nearly 46 million are without insurance entirely. It is a priority for the American people and a pillar of the new foundation we are seeking to build for our economy.

We'll continue to keep you posted about this and other important issues.

Thank you,

Barack Obama

P.S. If you'd like to get more in-depth information about health reform and how you can participate, be sure to visit http://www.HealthReform.gov .

Response:

Dear Mr. President:

Thank you for your email. I am in agreement with you when you state that we must change the way providers deliver health care in America today. Moreover, you have accurately articulated that the health care industry in general is raking in record revenues and profits for products and services that have become grossly inferior as evidenced by the highly publicized outcome statistics.

However, as a health professional and expert in patient safety and the quality of health care in institutional and home settings, I am deeply troubled with regard to the stated priorities of the proposed legislation and its implementation.

First, with all of the published materials disseminated over the last few months on proposed health care reform legislation, the issue of poor quality of care costing the lives of about 200,000 Americans per year seems to have been skipped over. The emphasis has been on the cost of care rather than on the fact that medical and nursing mistakes and negligence are the fifth leading cause of death in the United States today. Moreover, there are almost three times those many who suffer catastrophic injuries. The Centers for Medicare and Medicaid Services has identified twenty-eight complications arising out of negligence that occur repeatedly in every hospital in America. Those are called "never events" because all can agree that those events should never happen. Among those are injuries from falls, bedsores, medication errors, hospital acquired infections, failure to monitor clinical changes, surgical instruments and sponges left in body cavities, failure to provide sufficient oxygen during surgery, and the like. In fact, statistically speaking, a woman with breast cancer who checks into a hospital has a higher risk of dying from medical and/or nursing negligence than from the cancer.

Furthermore, given that most doctors, nurses and therapists go to work with the intention of first doing no harm, there has to be a logical reason why the same "never events" keep happening at every hospital and nursing facility in America. The answer is simple. There are major flaws in the infrastructure design. The reason for such defects is twofold; lack of standards and absence of personal accountability. You see, Mr. President, avoiding unnecessary mishaps is a responsibility that falls on the leadership within each health care organization. Unfortunately, the industry is self-regulating and without codified standards and accountability we continue to have chaos because we cannot expect people to impose any level of strictness on themselves.

Therefore, health care reform legislation must have provisions that will require professionals and business managers to adhere to standards promoting patient safety and impose criminal and civil penalties for willfully breaching such canons. Please remember that as you move Congress into action with your leadership that 23 people are losing their lives every hour unnecessarily because of health care mistakes, negligence or wanton neglect.

Second, although it may be gratifying on the one hand to see former opponents of health care reform capitulate, I am not so impressed. Those former opponents, who successfully lobbied against health care reform and universal coverage under the Clinton administration, are the reason why health care today is such a mess and a major cause of death in America. The fact that special interest groups such as the AMA, HMO's, AHA and others are now supporting your call for health care reform is highly suspect. This sudden change in attitude can only have been sparked by the economic collapse and massive unemployment which threatens to erode their base of paying customers.

Therefore, partnering with government under the new liberal banner and giving up some of the obscene profits seems the best way out of the new dilemma. However, there appears to be an underlying intent to lobby Congress to increase the number of covered individuals and provide money for preventive screening and obesity reduction without disturbing the status quo on the lack of standards and absence of accountability in how health care delivery is to be managed under the "reformed" system. Hence, Mr. President, I urge you to regard the new overtures from the current leaders of the major health care organizations with healthy skepticism.

In conclusion, I plead for our political leaders to understand that in order for our health care system to truly function as a system, there must be such codified standards that require staff people and their leaders in all of the thousands of hospitals and nursing facilities across America to behave exactly the same way in protecting the safety and well-being of their patients. Aside from the moral imperative of saving lives and avoiding injury, the favorable impact of having more than 300,000 people per year who will become able to return to productive lives, earning a living and paying taxes is obvious. That, Mr. President, is the change we need.

Respectfully yours,
Thomas A. Sharon, RN, MPH
Patient Safety and Health Care Quality Consultant

The Republican Alternative: Same Old Yadda

After the election of 2008, the then leaderless down-and-out Republican Party came out with their own legislative proposal on health care reform in a desperate attempt to upstage the Democrats. The GOP lawmakers were stroking themselves with an exercise in futility because they didn't even have enough votes to launch a filibuster. Although they had to try to do something to justify their empty and meaningless existence as politicians, this political buffoonery was like trying to melt an iceberg with a hair dryer, with no place to plug it in.

In any event, the GOP health reform plan, which was identical to the do nothing campaign rhetoric of John McCain that pushed him into a humiliating defeat, was unveiled in the aftermath of the 2008 election and included the following:
1. Creation of marketplaces to offer insurance choice. Make more private insurance options available to everyone without creating a public insurance system;
2. $2,290 tax credit per individual; $5,710 per family;
3. Investment in chronic disease prevention for diabetes, cancer, etc.
4. Medicare, Medicaid reform; will attempt to get people off of Medicaid and into private insurers;
5. Creation of independent health courts to resolve malpractice disputes outside the current system.

First, the creation of a market place to offer insurance choice wouldn't have changed anything. Private insurance options is what we have had all along and it's the principle reason why health care today is such a mess with organized criminals charging exorbitant prices for inferior products and services, rationing specialty care and gouging the public with ever-increasing prices. This mafia-style system was one of the main reasons why most of our manufacturing jobs got shipped to China and elsewhere with the automobile industry finding itself on the verge of total collapse. The health care debacle has been the driving force behind our sudden shift into a Stalinist Soviet style take-over of American industry, which I might add started under Republican President George W. Bush.

Second, the suggested tax credit of $2,290 for individuals and $5,710 per family is on par with what HMO's are currently charging for premiums with a $6,000 deductible. Therefore, the tax credit goes to the HMO and the consumer still has to pay the first $6,000 per year of medical expenses out of pocket. That's the big rip-off and the GOP wants to maintain the status quo while the HMO corporate executives have already been in the oval office kissing the ring of the new boss of bosses.

Third, suggesting investment for the prevention of chronic diseases such as "diabetes, cancer, etc." goes to show that the then defunct and partially rehabilitated GOP leaders are health-illiterates with nothing to offer. Moreover, the prevention of any avertable disease or complications there from rests with the affected individual because it requires changes in life style and behavior; and you can't legislate behavior modification and still call this a democracy.

Fourth, the suggestion to privatize Medicare and Medicaid as part of a new health care reform bill was mind-boggling because this had been ongoing for the last twenty years. Just about every Medicare recipient has had the option to join a private HMO and guess what? They're still not getting too many takers because the private plan puts the sick elderly in the hands of greedy profiteers and our seniors know it. The HMO's can't get more in premiums from the government, so they make their money by putting up confusing roadblocks to receiving specialist care and let the old folks die while corporate criminals enjoy Congressional immunity from civil and criminal prosecution. This scenario is reminiscent of the famous line in "Godfather Part II" from the character Hyman Roth when he spoke to Michael Corleone to entice him to invest two million dollars in Cuban enterprise under the corrupt Batista regime while it was crumbling under the Castro rebellion, "We finally have what we've always wanted—partnership with a government."

Fifth, the bid to create a health court to remove malpractice lawsuits from the court system is no surprise. The

Republicans have always advocated against victims of medical and nursing negligence, blaming their lawyers for all of it while the medical establishment continues to refuse to accept any responsibility. This proposal would allow the AMA to act as judge and jury for every negligence claim against a health care provider and give them absolute authority as to who may testify as an expert on behalf of the victim. Moreover, it's funny how the term "health court" popped up in the AMA's letter to President Obama. What's even funnier is that the Republican members of Congress are tripping over each other in their rush to kowtow to the AMA lobbists, while their client is licking the boots of the chief Democrat, President Obama.

Finally, there was no mention of quality of care and patient safety because the AMA won't allow it. Obviously, they want the health care industry to remain unregulated. The Democrats, on the other hand, at least paid some lip service to acknowledge that there are some issues with quality even though they don't have a viable plan for making health care safe.

Still, the Republicans want health care to remain as is, while the Democrats want to implement their socialist agenda with regard to taking control of the managed care industry making high tech care less available to the masses, make corporate profiteering less blatant and show a veneer of quality improvement while changing nothing in how providers deliver their services. Furthermore, the Republicans are marching in step with the insurance companies, the AMA and the AHA (American Hospital Association) while those former GOP congressional clients are rushing across the aisle and to the White House cajoling Democrat lawmakers and President Obama to let them continue feeding at the trough in exchange for their support. Such is politics. If Rod Serling were alive today, he would be telling us, "You have made a left turn off the map of reality and have entered the realm of chaotic imagination in the Twilight Zone."

What Happened to Patient Safety?

Amid all of the heated debates, blogs, press conferences, media releases and the like, I didn't see any mention of patient safety as the debates heated up in 2009. Not one lawmaker was even suggesting that we needed to save two hundred thousand lives per year. I felt like I was screaming from the roof tops and nobody was paying attention. What's more, I'm still screaming in 2012 and still no one is listening. Furthermore, most of those untimely preventable deaths are still occurring in all of our fine world class hospitals.

Therefore, since President Obama and the new Congress seemed to be willing to continue to let the hospital industry remain self-regulated as to patient safety, we need to take a look at how this was being done. In other words, what were the hospital executives, i.e. C.E.O's, C.N.O.'s (chief nursing officer) and their boards of directors doing in their respective institutions to minimize accidental death and catastrophic injuries? As we shall see, they are doing a lot but accomplishing nothing.

Since the scandalous revelation in 1999 by the Institute of Medicine of the pandemic of medical and nursing negligence, most hospitals have created a new job entitled "Patient Safety Officer" (PSO). They hired individuals like me on staff and some as outside consultants. So let's take a closer look at this activity by reviewing and analyzing a typical job description:

"The Patient Safety Specialist is responsible for planning, organizing, developing, managing, and evaluating a complex medical center patient safety program (HAP, BH, LTC, & HC

programs). This includes but is not limited to:
1. Developing and coordinating internal review systems to assure that clinical and administrative patient safety activities are in compliance with agency and accrediting standards and regulatory requirements;
2. Training and implementation of the Joint Commission National Patient Safety Goals, Root Cause Analysis and Health Care Failure Mode & Effects Analysis;
3. Reporting trend analysis and tracking to ensure follow-up for the facility's patient safety program activities."

First, we can see that from the perspective of hospital management, patient safety is complex and cumbersome with both clinical and administrative aspects. The system of regulation is fragmented and confusing with overlaps and conflicts. There are multiple government agencies providing regulatory oversight, such as health department, fire department, buildings department and the like with accreditation standards, professional association standards and regulatory codes from all the aforementioned departments. The internal review systems is an interesting nomenclature because while the PSO is reviewing charts to look at compliance issues, patients are falling out of bed, developing bedsores and being subjected to incompetence and neglect.

Second, the training and implementation of "Joint Commission National Patient Safety Goals, Root Cause Analysis and Healthcare Failure Mode & Effects Analysis" isn't working either. It's the same old ineffectual pseudo-intellectual mumbo jumbo. The bottom line is management and staff people have to learn how to think in a new paradigm like "Zero tolerance for patient falls, and bedsores". They need to stop using rhetoric like "Unfortunate but unavoidable" because it is a nefarious tool for avoiding accountability. Accidental patient death is the unintended consequence of accepting certain events that should never happen as being unavoidable.

Third, the job description of "reporting trend analysis and tracking to ensure follow-up for the facility's patient safety program activities" is the best way to insure that the untoward events that cause injury and death will keep happening repeatedly. That is another way of saying, "Take notes, tell your bosses what's going on, don't rock the boat and make it all look good to show the public that were doing something about patient safety. If there is any backlash, call it 'unfortunate but unavoidable'."

In brief, all of the above described fancy foot work is worthless because of the higher risk of death for people entering any hospital than from most of the diseases or injuries that they are seeking to treat. Therefore, in the highly publicized, hotly debated topic of health care reform, with major legislation purported to reduce health care spending, without some serious review and analysis of the hazards and horrors of hospital and nursing home care, truth in advertising laws should require health care institutions to have signs over their doors saying, "ENTER AT YOUR OWN RISK".

Patient Safety Awareness Week

The Lucian Leape Institute at the National Patient Safety Foundation, launched in 2007, functions as a think tank to define strategic paths and issue calls to action for the field of patient safety and is intended to provide vision and context for the many efforts underway within the health care system. This "think tank", which suddenly popped up during the Obama campaign invented "Patient Safety Awareness Week" in 2009 in their big effort to promote patient safety in a way that was guaranteed to fail.

After two years of "thinking", their big "call to action" was to publish a paraphrased standard "patient's bill of rights" that had been around for the last thirty plus years. Moreover, the foregoing is a list of promises not to engage in criminal acts of patient abuse, violation of HIPPA laws and violation of civil rights laws. There is nothing in this instrument that actually promised to focus on safety issues other than "We pledge to hold ourselves to the highest quality and safety standards." This vague reference to quality and safety standards was empty and meaningless because it did not specify what those standards are.

In retrospect, the "thinkers" should have been asking the health care institutional management teams and professional staff to accept responsibility and be accountable for their actions or lack thereof and provide a written guarantee to all consumers as follows:

1. "We promise not to let you fall;
2. We promise that only competent trained and supervised personal will perform invasive procedures on you;
3. We promise that if a student or intern has to do a procedure for the first time under appropriate supervision we will tell you and ask your permission;
4. We promise that you won't develop any bedsores because we will actually turn and reposition you if you need it and we will provide an appropriate pressure relieving mattress;
5. We promise that your nurse will act as your advocate to insure that you have access to competent medical care at all times;
6. We promise that we will inform you when the staffing level and nurse's workload become unsafe;
7. We promise that all medical equipment will be in good repair;

8. We promise that you will always get the right medication at the right time in the right dosage and the right route of administration;
9. We promise that we will protect you at all costs during surgery and you don't have to worry about going home with foreign objects inside your body;
10. We promise that we will properly identify you and the part of your body that requires surgery and that you will never have to undergo someone else's procedure;
11. We promise that we will never admit you to our facility unless there is an available bed so you won't have to stay in the emergency room for several days
12. We promise that if there are no available beds we will transfer you to the nearest appropriate facility for admission within 4 hours;
13. We promise never to serve scalding hot beverages or food;
14. We promise to monitor your food intake so that you won't choke to death;
15. We promise to monitor your unborn child for fetal distress and take appropriate action in a timely manner;
16. We promise that we will take only that amount of blood for testing that is required so that we never cause you to suffer from blood-loss anemia;
17. We promise that our nurses will always monitor your clinical condition and report changes immediately to your treating physician;
18. We promise to carry out doctors' orders in a timely fashion and refuse to carry out orders that are clearly not in your best interest;
19. We promise to inform you immediately when your nurse

has reservations about your treatment and let you know that you have the right to a second opinion before accepting any prescribed regimen;
20. We promise never to give you any medication or foods to which you are allergic;
21. We promise that if we screw up and you get hurt we will immediately provide complete disclosure, accept responsibility, beg for your forgiveness and offer fair compensation for the harm we caused."

Finally, it seemed bizarre that we had a "patient safety awareness week" while our law makers were proposing health care reform legislation with no awareness that patients had been unsafe. On the other hand, it is not clear just how NPSF defines "patient safety awareness". Does it mean raising public consciousness to become aware of how perilous health care has become so that consumers will realize the danger they're in when entering a hospital or nursing home? Or, perhaps it means that health care management personnel should become aware of what a lousy job they are doing in keeping their patient's safe. Then again, maybe it means that we should all have bombarded our congresspersons and senators with emails and phone calls telling them to include "patient safety awareness" while contemplating health care reform legislation.

Organized Medicine was ready to Deal

Comments on the Letter to President Obama from the Heads of the Six Families of Organized Medicine

President Obama had announced his goal of having

health care reform enacted by Congress by the end of the 2009 calendar year. However, in an effort to draw attention away from her flap with the C.I.A., Nancy Pelosi announced that she would have the bill on Obama's desk for signature by the end of July, which was not possible; unless the deal was already done. There were no Congressional hearings and no debates; there wouldn't even be any time for anyone to read the bill. This was the new rubber stamp congress at work.

The disconcerting part in this new political process was that with one party control of Capitol Hill, anything could happen. Things were unfolding so fast I felt like I was watching Saturday Night Live on C-Span. Assuming that Pelosi was only crazy and not stupid, the rapidity with which Congress could write such life-altering legislation with so much apparent confusion and debate, could lead to only one conclusion; the bill was already drafted before the election and all of the debate and discussion we were seeing was just for show. The agenda was set before the match, like TV wrestling. Otherwise, how did we get this letter to President Obama signed by the heads of the six families of organized medicine telling us what the new reformed health care industry was going to look like? Did they come up with all of these clever diabolical solutions from one meeting at the White House? Of course not! They had many meetings with Obama representatives and drafted their proposals long before they made public their willingness to cooperate. The irony was that these were the same people who fought against changing the status quo and engaged in price gouging for inferior products and services.

Therefore we need to hone in for a closer look at the letter to Obama, unravel the spin and smell what they have ben shoveling at us.

From Lip to Law

May 11, 2009
The President
The White House
Washington, D.C. 20500

Dear Mr. President:
We believe that all Americans should have access to affordable, high quality health care services. Thus, we applaud your strong commitment to reforming our nation's health care system. The times demand and the nation expects that we, as health care leaders, work with you to reform the health care system.

Without the spin: *We fought long and hard against socialized medicine, but now that the economy collapsed and everyone is going bankrupt we want to get our hands on some of that bailout money and protect our customer base so we can keep gouging them. So now we can have what we've always wanted, real partnership with a government.*

The annual growth in national health expenditures—including public and private spending—is projected by government actuaries to average 6.2% through the next decade. At that rate, the percent of gross domestic product spent on health care would increase from 17.6% this year to 20.3% in 2018—higher than any other country in the world.

Without the spin: *Oops! I guess you can't get blood from a turnip.*

We are determined to work together to provide quality, affordable coverage and access for every American. It is critical, however, that health reform also enhance quality, improve the overall health of the population, and reduce cost growth. We believe that the proper approach to

achieve and sustain reduced cost growth is one that will: improve the population's health; continuously improve quality; encourage the advancement of medical treatments, approaches, and science; streamline administration; and encourage efficient care delivery based on evidence and best practice.

Without the spin: If you pump some of those billions that you're throwing around into our companies we'll come up with more designer drugs, fancy gadgets, great catch-phrases that work and cut off some of the administrative fat. We'll talk to our people and make them an offer they can't refuse.

To achieve all of these goals, we have joined together in an unprecedented effort, as private sector stakeholders—physicians, hospitals, other health care workers, payers, suppliers, manufacturers, and organized labor—to offer concrete initiatives that will transform the health care system. As restructuring takes hold and the population's health improves over the coming decade, we will do our part to achieve your Administration's goal of decreasing by 1.5 percentage points the annual health care spending growth rate—saving $2 trillion or more. This represents more than a 20% reduction in the projected rate of growth. We believe this approach can be highly successful and can help the nation to achieve the reform goals we all share.

Without the spin: We'll knock 1.5% off our annual price increases so the cost of health care will go up by only 4.7% per year. The doctors won't take anymore pay cuts, but we can get the labor unions to eat it.

To respond to this challenge, we are developing consensus proposals to reduce the rate of increase in future health and insurance costs through changes made in all sectors of the health care system. We are committed to taking action in public-private partnership to create a more stable and sustainable health care system that will achieve billions in savings through:

Without the spin: Buy us out? We buy you out, you don't buy us out. Who do you think you're talking to? We made our bones when you were still going out with cheerleaders! How much did you have in mind?

Implementing proposals in all sectors of the health care system, focusing on administrative simplification, standardization, and transparency that supports effective markets;

Without the spin: It's time for some of our fat cats to bailout with their golden parachutes. We'll give them their bonuses and send them on their way.

• Reducing over-use and under-use of health care by aligning quality and efficiency incentives among providers across the continuum of care so that physicians, hospitals, and other health care providers are encouraged and enabled to work together towards the highest standards of quality and efficiency;

Without the spin: We'll decide who's getting too much and who needs more. We'll have to go pull some plugs to eliminate the inefficient use of resources. Sure we make mistakes; but we can bury them.

• Encouraging coordinated care, both in the public and private sectors, and adherence to evidence-based best practices and therapies that reduce hospitalization, manage chronic disease more efficiently and effectively, and implement proven clinical prevention strategies;

Without the spin: We'll get our doctors to toe the line and practice real medicine for a change. It's amazing what we can accomplish with a few billion dollars of bailout money.

• Reducing the cost of doing business by addressing

cost drivers in each sector and through common sense improvements in care delivery models, health information technology, workforce deployment and development, and regulatory reforms.

Without the spin: We'll cut down on some of those lavish meetings and conventions, you give us the 20 billion dollars that Congress set aside for health information technology and we'll get our workforce to take some pay cuts.

These and other reforms will make our health care system stronger and more sustainable. However, there are many important factors driving health care costs that are beyond the control of the delivery system alone. Billions in savings can be achieved through a large-scale national effort of health promotion and disease prevention to reduce the prevalence of chronic disease and poor health status, which leads to unnecessary sickness and higher health costs. Reform should include a specific focus on obesity prevention commensurate with the scale of the problem.

Without the spin: You've got a sedentary, fast-food eating, overweight, aging population sucking in poison gasses. What do you want us to do about that? You might consider getting your Congress to pass an obesity tax and charge by the pound.

These initiatives are crucial to transform health care in America and to achieve our goal of reducing the rate of growth in health costs. We, as stakeholder representatives, are committed to doing our part to make reform a reality in order to make the system more affordable and effective for patients and purchasers. We stand ready to work with you to accomplish this goal.

Without the spin: Okay, maybe we did go a tad too far with our price gouging practices, shabby services and toxic drugs. So we're willing to cut

Uncle Sam in as a partner for a measly few hundred billion. What do you say? It's a good business.

Sincerely,

Stephen J. Ubl
President and CEO
Advanced Medical
Technology Association

Rich Umbdenstock
President and CEO
American Hospital
 Association

Billy Tauzin
President and CEO
Pharmaceutical
Research
 and Manufacturers of
America

Karen Ignagni
President and CEO
America's Health
 Insurance Plans

J. James Rohack, MD
President-elect
American Medical
 Association

Dennis Rivera
Chair, SEIU
Healthcare
Service Employees
 International Union

In conclusion, it is easy to see that the politicians have to follow the recommendations of the heads of the six families of organized medicine. Otherwise, how would the lawmakers know where to start? Therefore we can conclude that health care reform, as it was called, will never include patient safety. Certainly there will be more organized delivery for those who are currently uninsured, but we cannot expect to reduce the risk of being killed by our health care providers unless there are some public congressional hearings to uncover the root causes of so many preventable deaths per year.

Wrap Up

Quality of care does not depend on who pays for it or how much a doctor makes. It depends on the attitudes and behaviors of millions of health care workers and the kind of leadership they have. It's a daunting task indeed that requires professional re-education on how to take their responsibility seriously because lives hang in the balance.

Finally, it was laughable to see the very leaders responsible for the mess come to the White House lunch table to make recommendations for health care reform. It's like listening to bank robbers making recommendations to improve security.

In brief, after reviewing the rhetoric that went through weekly transformations for more than a year, we begin to gain the clarity to see the manipulations through a massive dog-and-pony show to make us believe that our elected officials were acting in our best interest, when in reality the entire process was the unfolding of a conspiracy to create chaos and promote the population reduction of seniors; forcing the elderly to accept death without using costly health care resources.

10. The Political Pretext

Although there was a lot of rhetoric coming from the Obama camp about improving the quality of health care, the powerful lobby of the six families of organized medicine quickly headed off any effort to put patient safety legislation into reality. The heads of the six families made very clear that they were not going to take responsibility for killing more than a million people since 9/11/2001.

Thus, there would be no health care reform in the real sense because the leaders of organized medicine would first have to admit that their constituents' methods needed reforming. Therefore, they invented catch phrases and buzzwords to create the illusion that they were proposing new ways of delivering health care services, so that quality of care issues need not be addressed through legislation. The Obama administration and congressional leaders quickly rolled over because having a cooperative arrangement with the health care professionals and institutions would allow government officials to impose command and control over utilization of health care products and services.

Fighting the Wrong Battles

Right about mid-2009, there seemed to be a glitch in the Senate; Senator Ted Kennedy, shortly before his death, and Senator Baucus were having a raucous debate about how to set up health care reform in the new America. According to news media reports, the two Democratic Senate leaders were at odds about whether to continue to have HMO's competing in an insurance exchange or just cover everyone from birth to death under a unified Federal Government health insurance plan

(NHIP). The two Senators appeared to be back-peddling to try to snooker the public into thinking that there was no disagreement. Too late; we knew better. Of course any hint of disunity among the all-powerful democrats would have lead us ordinary citizens to believe that maybe there wouldn't be a bill ready for President Obama to sign by August 1, 2009 as Speaker Nancy Pelosi had promised before the world.

However, the flap over whether government or a mix of competing corporate criminal types should control the delivery of health care products and services could only be a legitimate issue if one could argue how either proposal would impact favorably on improving quality. The big question as yet unanswered was, "How do we eliminate the careless mistakes that continue to kill people at such an alarming rate?" If we wanted to compare private industry with government as providers of health care coverage, we could have done that because we have had both systems in place for decades. The truth is, they both suck.

The private sector is guilty of price gouging and swindling their customers out of getting competent medical care. The Federal Government is guilty of setting up a bureaucratic morass reducing physician income and creating a confusing maze of paper work to set up roadblocks against reimbursement, while preventing patients from getting medical equipment and supplies with unreasonable denials. Moreover, since government uses private insurance to act as intermediaries, the final result is the same for the public and private sectors.

Meanwhile, nobody can go into a hospital without risking death from sloppy health care delivery. Therefore, because the new health care reform act was not going to reform the government in eliminating the congressional pork, we got more of the same. Congress can pass a bill, but the implementation of it is a different matter. Therefore, the question of who will pay the providers for their services and products should be answered first. More importantly however, Congress should have been looking for ways to codify patient safety standards and provide funding for enforcement.

The Pretext Proposals

The first bill for health care reform, H.R. 676, was on the floor of the House of Representatives ready for the great debate by the end of the first quarter of 2009. Opponents of single payer health care wanted to sweep it off the floor into the Congressional trash bin. This seemed to be the only remaining controversy, since nobody cared about patient safety. However, the new bill, although it smelled like a watered down version of Hillary Clinton's colossal failure, had some elements in it that did address quality issues. Also the fact that this bill proposed to vaporize the for-profit HMO's and to transform the entire health care provider industry into non-profit organizations seemed inherently appealing because on the surface, at least, it struck at the heart of the whole problem with health care being a price-gouging, profiteering, collusive oligopoly with no interest in consumer satisfaction and safety. However, my one big reservation was with the implementation. The new bill called for establishing a huge bureaucracy and hiring all of the HMO personnel who would become jobless because of H.R. 676. The scariest part of the proposed legislation was that it employed the same HMO buzz words, like "medically necessary". Although H.R. 676 never made it to a vote, an analysis of what it contained serves as a clue to understanding the nefarious agenda of the government imposing its socialist will on who shall live and who shall die.

Eligibility

The eligibility requirement was simple enough—every human being on American soil would get a health card. The application would never ask for a social security number, so obviously all illegal aliens would be able to join. It kind of made sense because we've been paying for their care anyway; we might as well do it for a lot less in clinics and doctors' offices rather than in emergency rooms. On the other hand, there was one huge problem with this type of open enrollment; the national health card would be an open invitation for millions more to sneak across the borders to get free American-style health care service.

Benefits

The proposed health care reform bill H.R. 676 contained the most comprehensive benefits I had ever seen, with home care, medical equipment and supplies, alternative medicine, long term care, dental, hearing aids and vision correction (excluding laser treatment). The national health insurance card would be accepted in all provider facilities throughout the United States so that portability would no longer have been an issue and there would not be any out-of-pocket costs to the insured. Moreover, the only exclusions were cosmetic dentistry and surgery which left open the question as to how to define "cosmetic."

Qualification of Participating Providers

For profit hospitals and nursing homes would be out of business with the government compensating the proprietors, partners and/or shareholders for all tangible assets confiscated in the process. All institutional health care providers would be required to be non-profit organizations. Quality of care would then be part of the qualification process with safe staffing and other quality guidelines. The section on patient safety and quality would need to become the crucial element of any new health reform law. However, unless it was more clearly defined it would become nothing more than useless rhetoric with the providers left to self-regulate as usual and continue to cause death and injury on a gargantuan scale.

Destruction of the HMO's

Obliterating the HMO's seemed to be the best part of this new plan. However, the management and operations personnel who would be displaced from their jobs would become government employees and would run the back office operations of the new national health insurance plan (NHIP). The insurance companies would no longer be allowed to provide any health care coverage. Although getting rid of the HMO's was tempting, the prospect of turning profiteers into bureaucrats was scary.

Moreover, if the government replaces the for-profit HMO's with itself using the same cost-cutting methodology, we consumers would be back in the same situation—victimized by denial of life-saving health care with no legal recourse. We cannot expect a sudden outpouring of human compassion simply because the corporate criminals become government officials.

In conclusion, the total comprehensive benefit package was certainly attractive, but found to be impractical because the cost would be three hundred percent greater than the total tax revenue of the all levels of government. Additionally, the drafters of the new health care reform legislation failed to take a serious look at the miserable failure of government run health care institutions and third party payment systems like Medicare and Medicaid. With a single party system, if Congress couldn't learn by the mistakes of our past and present, they would only accomplish taking a fragmented world of chaos and shoving it all under one roof, broken down by regions, states and localities. The only spark of hope in H.R. 676 was the brief mention of quality and safety standards. If Congress could focus on the safety aspect in an appropriate manner with a benefit package available to all on a sliding scale premium charge based on income, the question of single or multi payer would be moot.

HELP!!!

It's hard to believe that we actually have had a United States Senate committee on health, education, labor and pensions (HELP) because the health system is in chaos, education is in the sewer with public school teachers being arrested for downloading child pornography in classrooms, labor has run amok and bankrupted the auto industry after chasing most manufacturing jobs overseas and pension funds have been decimated by the robber barons of wall street. It is even more maddening when you read the committee's mission statement on health.

"**The HELP Committee jurisdiction encompasses most of the agencies, institutes, and programs of the Department of Health and Human Services, including the Food and Drug Administration, the Centers for Disease Control and Prevention, the National Institutes of Health, the Administration on Aging, the Substance Abuse and Mental Health Services Administration, and the Agency for Healthcare Research and Quality. The Committee also oversees public health and health insurance statutes to** address emerging threats and changing patterns in the healthcare industry."

What we have seen here is a colossal failure—Congressional politics at its best. These are the lawmakers under the leadership of Senator Ted Kennedy who had oversight of the whole enchilada for several decades. In other words, they watched while the health care system continued to kill 200,000 people, year after year and never lifted a finger to investigate why. So which of the "enumerable threats and changing patterns in the health care industry" did the esteem committee address? After looking over the list of hearings and bills churned out of the HELP committee chambers, there was not one word about patient safety with 2 million people being killed from 2000 to 2010 because of medical and nursing negligence! They could have saved hundreds of thousands of lives by conducting emergency hearings on the root causes of preventable patient deaths and writing the appropriate legislation requiring standards for patient safety in health care like Congress has for passenger safety in the airlines. This HELP committee has more innocent blood on their hands than the Islamic terrorists we are supposed to be fighting.

To wit, we have the announcement of the last health care reform proposal that came from the HELP committee. I shall present this information and provide some responsive comments.

The key points of the HELP committee sanctions include the following:

"Assuring reliable, high-quality, affordable health insurance for all, including making available the option of a public plan."

What is reliable, high-quality, affordable health insurance? What does high-quality health insurance look like? Does that mean an insurance company that pays legitimate claims in a timely manner? When has that ever happened? Moreover, when has an insurance company ever been reliable about anything besides sending out invoices for premiums? On the other hand, the one thing we can rely on from all health insurers is to tell us that our doctors' recommendations are not medically necessary even if our lives depend on them.

Creating a higher quality, more efficient delivery system, including implementation of strategies to reduce hospital readmissions.

First you have to get the higher quality, more efficient delivery system to stop killing people at the rate of 23 per hour. Hospital readmission was never an issue for those 200,000 victims per year because they're dead.

Promoting prevention and wellness.

Now there's an original idea! Did the senators think that one up all by themselves, or did they have HELP?

Financing long-term services and support to ensure that vulnerable populations have access to meaningful, affordable coverage.

How about taking a look at all of the elder abuse and the massive amount of bedsores and other horrible injuries from gross neglect that runs rampant in most of the nursing homes across America? Take a look at the survey data on http://Medicare.gov. Oh, I forgot; Medicare is under the finance committee so there's no HELP for Medicare.

Investing in efforts to fight health care fraud and abuse.

What about all of the money spent on fighting health care fraud and abuse over the last fifty years? Has the illustrious committee ever accomplished anything other than photo ops and hot air?

Establishing shared responsibility between individuals, employers, insurers, and providers, and paying appropriately and fairly for reform.

What shared responsibility? Individuals have to learn how to avoid falling victim to medical and nursing negligence. Employers are interested bystanders who benefit from reduced sick calls and fewer untimely deaths, but do not have any responsibility in health care delivery. Insurers have to stop their price gouging and interfering with the doctor-patient relationships. Providers have to adhere to reasonable safety standards and take an authentic interest in their patient's safety and well-being. Each group has its own area of responsibility with a common interest. However, to call it "shared responsibility" was absurd.

One would have to conclude that empty words of stupidity have value if they serve the agenda of leaving the status quo as a matter of convenience in hatching a plan to take control of a chaotic health care delivery system that is already killing more people that the diseases being treated. Then it will be easier to decide who shall live and who shall die among the baby boomers of America.

As a follow up regarding the HELP committee, I have one big question for them. What did they do over the last eleven years to investigate the fact that health care providers had become the fifth leading cause of deaths in America? Shortly after the scandalous report of the Institute of Medicine in 1999, the Journal of the American Medical Association published an article that revealed the actual number of deaths due to health care negligence exceeded 225,000 per year with the following

breakdown[23]:
1. 106,000 patients die each year from the negative effects of medication
2. 80,000 patients die each year due to complications from infections incurred in hospitals
3. 20,000 deaths per year occur from other hospital errors
4. 12,000 people die every year as a result of unnecessary surgery
5. 7,000 medical malpractice deaths per year are attributed to medication errors in hospitals

Moreover, Institute of Medicine of the National Academies (IOM), the government agency that revealed the first scandalous hospital mistake death toll in 1999, reported 7 years later in 2006 that medication errors alone were causing reportable injuries to about 1.5 million people every year in all health care settings combined.

To sum up, experts in the field of patient safety know the root causes of so much mayhem and how to prevent it. Therefore, we as concerned citizens need to ask what President Obama and the new Congress are doing to address the issue of not having sufficient standards of safety in health care settings. Health care negligence is now declared by many sources to be the third leading cause of death in America topped only by heart disease and some cancers. So tell us, Mr. President and esteemed members of Congress, if, heaven forbid, any of you or your loved ones became victims of negligent health care, would you worry about who is going to pay for it?

---

[23] Journal of the American Medical Association; 2000 Jul 26;284(4):483-5

The Move from Health Care Reform to Health Insurance Reform

After months of debating there was still no word on patient safety from Congress. The Finance and HELP committees were still hammering and yammering about their respective versions of the Senate bill. The news hounds and talking heads were telling us that the big debate was still over single versus multi-payer health insurance and how we the people were going to pay the premiums despite the political rhetoric about drastic cost cutting measures. Tax the rich, the smokers, fatties and so on. Yet there was still no discussion about patient safety standards and the AMA was fiercely lobbying against finding fault with the quality of care. The SEIU, the largest health care labor union in America, has led many fights against management about maintaining safe staffing levels, but Dennis Rivera, the SEUI president, sat in that meeting with President Obama and the heads of the other five families of organized medicine and signed the follow-up letter that said nothing about patient safety. It was disheartening to watch this longtime labor leader and proponent of health care quality participate in such a shameful charade.

Moreover, cost containment was another big issue being promulgated by the Obama administration. The President wanted to lower the cost of acquiring health care coverage but anything short of a complete government takeover meant that he had to intercede with the private HMO's and force them to deflate their premiums. However, after nationalizing General Motors, and being criticized by Chavez and Castro for being too much of a left wing radical, President Obama shied away from a single party system. Therefore, he will have to pounce on the HMO's to back off from their price gouging and make some drastic cuts, leaving them on shaky ground. This was risky because the entire managed care infrastructure was built on the backs of the consumers with recommended procedures, equipment and supplies being arbitrarily and capriciously denied. Consequently, a reversal of price trends and the desperate greed for more profits will translate to more criminal behavior in denying paid-for benefits and blackmailing primary care physicians to treat conditions beyond their training and expertise.

Thus the Obama initiatives to decrease utilization, streamline the management of chronic disease and force HMO's to cut administrative overhead were doable as long as quality would remain a non-issue. What was this? But Obama said that he was going to do it all while improving quality. Pundits argued that all of the above factors would make health care delivery more efficient, which was an oxymoron because the people who deliver health care have been killing 200,000 of their customers every year. How was President Obama going to improve quality by throwing less money at an industry that had already performed so badly? Actually, there would have been a way to do it if by some miracle he had listened to the voices in the wilderness and propose that Congress include codified patient safety standard.

Alas, but the President did not answered any of my emails as of this date, so I had no way of knowing whether he would ever know about the above suggestion. As long as the Obama administration was going to remain oblivious to patient safety, they had to rename the "health care reform" effort and call it "health insurance reform."

The Obama Sell-out

In May of 2009 the State of California Department of

Public Health decided to make an example of two hospitals by levying fines of $25,000 each for using a faulty respirator on a man with emphysema, and sending a patient home after back surgery with a sponge stuffed in around his spine. Additionally, they levied lesser fines of varying amounts against eleven other hospitals for lapses in patient care that placed patients in jeopardy. Thus we have the same tire old methods with health department inspectors conducting surprise audits of patient cases once every three years on average and levying fines which rarely go above $25,000.

Now that the public eye was on health care reform, many state regulatory agencies were scurrying about to assess the damages. Many state health department officials added reporting requirements and removed the veil of secrecy from the realm of in-hospital negligence in hopes that the humiliation of bad publicity would motivate administrators to run a tighter ship. Thus far, we have seen no evidence that this strategy has ever worked. Nobody wanted to deal with the fact that there is a 1 in 500 risk of death just from being in any hospital even though that would be like an airliner falling out of the sky every week. However, if there were that much trouble with air travel, people have other options; whereas if someone is on the way to a hospital with a life-threatening condition, there is no other alternative.

Accordingly, what we need to realize is that the current regulation systems are utterly useless because there is no personal accountability other than becoming defendants in a medical malpractice lawsuit. For example, what do we do about a hospital corporate management team that blatantly refuses to keep its life support equipment in good repair? What if somebody dies because a machine doesn't work at the moment the staff needs to use it to correct a life-threatening condition? In any other situation, a person who knowingly causes and allows a potentially lethal condition to exist is guilty of criminally negligent homicide. If the situation were truly horrendous, the authorities might even ad "with depraved indifference". Therefore, every time a hospital administrator causes death with a wanton disregard for the patients' safety and well-being by refusing to provide equipment in good working order, that person should go to jail.

But that doesn't happen in this country because we don't have special safety standards like we have with air travel. A couple of years ago, when two pilots showed up drunk at a Texas airport there was a huge scandal and the inebriated flyboys never made it to the cockpit because they were arrested at the gate. When a surgeon shows up plastered, the operating room manager either cancels his cases for that day, or the good drunken doctor stands by and watches while a resident performs the procedure. There is usually no scandal and no disciplinary proceeding because the hospital business managers see the physician as their cash cow and they don't want to tarnish their public image.

In conclusion, President Obama kept saying through his campaign and the first six months of his presidency that the health care system was broken and that it was not sustainable. He claimed that we kept on paying more for less. Ironically, he was right; but he had changed his focus to coverage and cost and had decided not to deal with what goes on in hospitals, rehab centers and nursing homes with the more than 200,000 preventable deaths and more than 600,000 disabling injuries per year from trauma, pressure ulcers, medication errors, surgical blunders, infections, pulmonary emboli, internal hemorrhage and the like. It is really a simple matter of nurses, doctors and management personnel being more meticulous in how they maintain patient safety. There are certain procedures that they must perform at the beginning of every shift like checking equipment and supplies, assessing the patients and their environments and re-checking patients' identities.

However, health care workers are not diligent enough in conducting such procedures. If they were, there wouldn't be so many casualties. There are too many people in the health care professions and management who don't know how to promote patient safety and don't care to learn. Therefore, we needed Congress to develop a complete set of regulations requiring interventions for prevention of all of the named events that should never happen. Pilots are diligent in their safety checks because their lives are on the line too. Doctors and nurses need to have the same motivation for the same level of thoroughness; they need to have something to lose if they cause death or catastrophic injury through wanton negligence, like their livelihood and freedom.

End-of-Life Counselling

During July of 2009, some low-life nameless vermin among the denizens of Capitol Hill proposed that the new health care reform bill contain a mandate that all seniors 65 years of age or older must report for end-of-life counseling. There is absolutely no humanitarian benefit in doing this to our senior population and there is no financial benefit to the health care system unless this is an insidious plot to establish a euthanasia program to murder people in lieu of paying the increasing health care costs that comes with growing older. This depraved scheme instantly begged a few questions and comments.

First, I had to wonder why our society considers age 65 to

be the crossing point to the end of life. Who decided that people have to retire at that age anyway? My mother, Frances Ginsberg, of blessed memory, who recently passed away at 98, had decided at age 62 that she needed to start going to college, so she became a college graduate at 65 and went on for her masters and took that one two years later. Then she entered the work force starting a new career teaching seniors how to live productive lives. Then at age 75 she decided that it was time for her to go for career advancement and she started to work on her doctorate in psychology. Finally at age 80 she went back to Hungary and completed her doctorate at the University of Budapest. On the day of her graduation, the Chancellor handed her the diploma with an apology for the prior decades of their anti-Semitic policy of rejecting applications from Jewish students and professors.

Second, how would anyone have the skills to counsel another person on how to prepare for death? Does the government have any employees who died and came back to tell us what we can expect?

Third, when my mother returned from Hungary with her doctorate, we asked her, "So now that you have a PhD in psychology, what are you going to do with it?"

She replied, "I will now counsel young people on how to lead more productive lives."

We then asked her, "How old are all these young people?"

"Oh, about 65 or 70."

To my mother, being elderly was not a matter of biological age; it was a matter of one's personal level of productivity. Accordingly, I have to say that this notion of mandating end-of-life counseling at age 65 as part of the health care reform act is probably the most diabolical idea that anyone has ever put forth. Although seeing how our leaders in Congress have been performing lately, as flabbergasting as it was, this latest wave of insidiousness was not surprising.

In conclusion, I keep having this mental image of what I would see if I were a giant and suddenly lifted up the dome of the Capitol building to let in the sunshine; I would see hundreds of denizens on both sides of the aisle scurrying about to hide in the shadows.

The Barking Blue Dogs Buried their Bones

The 111th Congress reconvened on or about September 7, 2009, and they certainly had a fight on their hands. Although notwithstanding that the Speaker gloated over the fact that the Republicans were virtually invisible since the asses became fleas on the elephants, the fight seemed to be between the autocratic Democratic Socialist hags from the Left Coast and the fine people of the United States of America. Even Dorothy from Kansas couldn't make the wicked witch of the West (WWW) melt away. Moreover, regarding the good old barking "Blue Dogs", the WWW was telling the press that she had thrown them a couple of bones to bury and taught them a few new tricks, so they wouldn't be a problem. They were also house broken and had no teeth.

Therefore, the only things that stood in the way of Obama's public option, according to Madame Speaker, were the Nazi skinhead thugs that were invading the town hall meetings and trying to intimidate the esteemed members of Congress into voting no. The only problem I was having with her descriptive hyperbole was that I had not seen any Nazi skinhead thugs at any of the televised town hall meetings. I have only seen average

American citizens of all ages and from all occupations and life styles, with elderly and disabled among them expressing their outrage at a Congress that votes a 1000-page bill into law without reading a single word merely because Obama and Pelosi said to do so, as if they were following the word of G-d. The constituents were actually saying, "You morons don't work for Obama and Pelosi, you work for us!"

Nonetheless, the big argument narrowed to whether or not the Federal Government should start its own HMO to compete with the private sector, like FedEx and UPS versus the United States Post Office, as President Barack Obama had pointed out. Of course, on the surface, this analogy made sense because if anyone who wasn't brain dead and needed to have a package delivered by a reliable carrier, he or she would never trust the bureaucrats at the Post Office. Thus, the private carriers, who charge more, rely on the need for reliable, efficient customer service to stay in business.

However, the problem with Obama's argument is that reliability and efficiency in health care, public or private, is fantasy. The people who still believe in the third biggest lie, "We have the best health care in the world," are living in a fool's paradise. The reality check is that health care is neither reliable nor efficient, for even the super wealthy and high ranking government officials are subject to the same medical mistakes that kill so many people per year. The only possible exception is Obama, who smugly stated that he has a doctor following him wherever he goes like a faithful hound. Then again, even the President's personal lapdog physician can screw around with patient safety and who's going to know?

Therefore, the big missing piece of this entire jigsaw puzzle is the fact that the "best in the world" American health care system had become the third leading cause of death in the United States. In that context, the Democrats will not be doing the 46 million uncovered Americans such a big favor until they start addressing the need for legislated basic patient safety standards with criminal penalties for any licensed health professional whose betrayal of the public trust causes catastrophic injury and death. In conclusion, while our health care system remains so dangerous all arguments over who is going to be running the show are moot.

Who Shall Live and Who Shall Die?

One of the frightening aspects of moving into a Reformed Health Care System is the prospect of rationing. There are a number of articles by and about Dr. Ezekiel Emanuel, who has become the principle adviser to Barack Obama on his health care policy. As a bioethicist, Dr. Emanuel has written extensively on the issue of how to allocate lifesaving medical treatment when there isn't enough to save all those who have a good chance for survival. Currently, doctors and administrators find themselves faced with the question of who should live and who should die with organ transplantation. For every available heart, kidney and liver, there are more than a few eligible recipients. Who gets to make the final choice among multiple candidates for any particular organ and what criteria do they use to make their selections? Moreover, this problem will grow exponentially in the next fifteen years when the average age of the baby boomer generation reaches to the mid-seventies. There will be about thirty patients in critical condition for every intensive care unit bed requiring an average nurse-to-patient ratio of 1:2. Although hospitals can easily convert regular floor rooms into intensive care units, finding enough nurses to staff them is another story because we don't have enough to take care of the patient loads we have now.

Thus, we would do well to heed the warnings of Dr. Emanuel when he says that we will need to establish criteria for who should receive lifesaving treatment when demand exceeds supply. However, to reduce such a deep philosophical and ethical question to mere statistical analysis based on age and potential contribution to society is dangerously void of compassion and opens the door to the euthanasia practiced by the medical establishment of Nazi Germany. The main problem with Dr. Emanuel's proposals is that the power over deciding who shall die and who shall live cannot legitimately rest with any single human or panel group.

Emanuel believes that doctors should have the discretion to withhold medical treatment from people who do not meet some arbitrary criteria for potential contribution to society loosely based on age and survival probability. But suppose those numbers are equal for a particular group of patients and the choice has to be further narrowed. Will they choose the scientist over the fireperson? What if the scientist invents a new type of germ warfare and the device kills one hundred million people? Wouldn't society be better off with the fireperson who runs into a burning building to save lives? The main point is that everyone wants to live and the government does not have the authority according to our constitution to deprive its citizens of the right to life, liberty and the pursuit of happiness without due process. Of course there are exceptions during times of extreme emergency when the authorities have to take certain measures to protect the common good as in setting up triage during disasters to decide medical priority on the likelihood of survival. However, a patient walking into a doctor's office or even going to the emergency room by ambulance does not qualify for disaster protocol. Thus, to deny people access to life saving treatment because they don't fit in a statistical category would require a callous and depraved indifference to human life.

Consequently, we already have occasional situations in which someone has to make a choice between two or more candidates for a life-saving treatment. The only viable criterion for such a choice is who is the most likely to die while waiting. At best it is only guess work, but the person in power has to be satisfied that the decision to provide lifesaving treatment to one does not necessarily mean certain death for the others. Thus, to empower anyone to make a decision based on arbitrary criteria to cause death by withholding lifesaving measures opens the door to another Holocaust.

Figures Lie and Liars Figure in the Class War

The fantasy that we have the best health care system in the world is a perfect example of how figures lie and liars figure. The conservative pundits are extolling the virtues of the current state of health care by quoting statistics published in Lancet in 2008[24] showing that breast cancer survival rates are higher in the United States than in Great Britain and the rest of Europe; 83.9%, 69.7% and 73.1% respectively. However, this is where people can use statistics to mislead the public into thinking that we need not disturb the status quo. If you look at our health care system you will see that it has three tiers; private insurance, Medicaid and Medicare, and uninsured. The study published in

---

[24] Lancet Oncology; 2008 Aug;9(8):730-56.

the Cancer Journal for Clinicians[25] showed a differential in survival rates from breast and colorectal cancer according to insurance status among other variables. The survival rate for those with private insurance is 78% as opposed to 67% and 65% respectively for Medicaid and the uninsured. This stands to reason as those with private insurance are generally better informed and have more access to early screening procedures than the Medicaid and the uninsured population.

Therefore, on the one hand, the above statistical advantage for the privately insured decry the arguments for setting up the "public option" as a means for achieving the ultimate goal of socialized health care in the United States. It is painfully obvious that about half of our population enjoy health care that is apparently superior to the systems in England and Canada while the other half are worse off than their European and north-of-the-border counterparts. Thus this whole debate for and against the Obama care plan has turned into a class warfare struggle of those with the private coverage against those without and it's getting uglier by the day. The Republicans and independent conservatives claim that if we let the rest of the population into the private insurance club that they will become worse off because the waiting rooms and appointment schedules will be too crowded.

On the other hand, however, from the perspective of the bottom half of the population who are either government-dependent or uninsured, things can't get any worse. Access to screening for early detection of cancer and other preventive medicine modalities is just not there. Moreover, doctors who accept Medicaid and Medicare receive so little pay compared to

---

[25] Cancer J Clin. 2008; 58:9-31

private HMO compensation that they have to depend on high volume. This payless assembly line medicine must logically result in less time per patient causing a higher incidence of misdiagnoses and other blunders. Certainly the more time a doctor spends listening to a patient's concerns, the better the outcome. Medical students learn early on that fifty percent of the diagnostic accuracy comes from taking a precise medical and social history.

In conclusion, it is obvious from the information that we have at hand that government-run health care when compared to the private sector is a dismal failure in this country. Thus, we can see the logic in arguing that a new federal system whereby all health care workers become Federal employees will pull the upper half of the population down rather than elevating the bottom. Nonetheless, there is still a dire need to improve the status of those 150 million Medicaid recipients and uninsured languishing without proper health care and it is entirely doable. What we need is for politicians to stop using the health care reform movement for personal advantage and get down to what this country's economy needs to get back on its feet; eliminate price gouging, put a stop to arbitrary denials of prescribed treatments, equalize compensation for physicians and other providers, cut administrative costs and improve patient safety by setting mandatory standards.

Wrap Up

We have seen the context of the health care debate turn on a dime from quality to coverage issues. The whole massive paper blizzard in congress was about whether to get rid of the private health insurance providers immediately or later. The

Congress decided on later to get past the resistance against a government single-payer system. Now that the Supreme Court has struck down mandatory health plan purchase, the private health coverage carriers will fold because they cannot survive selling health plans exclusively to a high risk population. As said previously, in order for a private HMO to survive it must sell plans into a population in which the healthy people are paying for the sick. Thus, if an HMO were to sell their health plans only to sick people it cannot survive because the premiums would not even cover a fraction of the cost.

Therefore, patient safety became an orphan. Nobody wants to own it because the political agenda is to grab control of health care with the blessings of the professional organizations. Any loss of public confidence in doctors and hospitals would lead to discovering the real mess that health care in America has become.

11. The Death Panel Shell Game

Something for Everyone

President Barack Obama made a smart political move in his "chicken-in-every-pot" health care reform speech in September of 2009. The smoke and mirrors with the thousands of pages of confusion, being an unprecedented move toward a national socialist health care autocracy, had failed. We the people had spoken out, declaring these Congressional proposals to be un-American. Hence, in a frenzied reaction to avoid political suicide Obama had to denounce arguments that the government was gearing up for euthanizing high cost health care patients as bogus; even in the face of Democrat proposals that would mandate end-of-life counseling for people over the age of sixty-five. He also denied that this health care reform movement was about government gaining control over people's private lives with access to centrally computerized health care records.

Additionally, the President addressed all of the arguments against the then current bills saying that this won't add a penny to the budget deficit because it will pay for itself. Those that have coverage can keep their status quo intact and those that don't' will have cheaper premiums and smaller deductibles; and everyone will have a "public option" with less bureaucracy, lower cost and better service. Obama even addressed the issue of medical malpractice causing doctors to drive up the cost of health care by practicing defensive medicine. He even said that Congress will look at things like "patient safety issues." Say what?

Finally, Obama said that when health insurance becomes affordable it has to be mandatory; but in the same breath he identified that there will still be a segment of the population—the people falling between the cracks—that won't be able to pay premiums. For those unfortunate souls, let there be Republican tax credits. All of the above is well and good—something for everybody with a promise to look into patient safety at some more convenient time while the carnage continues unabated. for

In summary, President Barack Obama did a good job claiming to be all inclusive with some yielding toward the Republican mind set. However, we have yet to see the impact of the shadow government of communist tinhorn dictators appointed as Czars of various categories like, car manufacturing, banking, green jobs, health care and the like. We are also still waiting for the formation of armed civilian enforcement troops that are supposed to become more powerful than the regular military; like the brown shirted guys who, in 1933, began attacking the Jewish communities in Germany; and the government paid thugs who recently bludgeoned to death a young woman in the streets of Teheran for speaking out in protest against the Iranian president. The only thing we don't have is a sincerity meter to know whether Obama is truly bowing to the will of the people or just tabling for the present a more clandestine long-term national socialist agenda.

The Veil of Secrecy

After Senator Baucus and his Democrat colleagues took a beating in the court of public opinion regarding all of their health care reform proposals, in October of 2009, they decided to change their strategy of openness to a veil of secrecy. This was the Senators' response to the public outcry against the placing of our future health, safety and well-being in the hands of the denizens of Capitol Hill; write a new bill and don't show it to anyone. Just take it to the floor for a vote after team Obama works on throwing the "blue dogs" a few bones.

However, as we have come to expect, the best kept secrets of the D.C. politicians always wind up on the six O'clock News. Baucus' new secret health care reform bill was no exception. The conservative pundits on Fox News were telling us that Baucus eliminated the "public option" and set up the new bill so that we have to pay in advance for benefits that won't kick in for at least two years. What happened to "we can't afford to wait because people are dying?" Moreover, to the delight of the American Medical Association (AMA) leadership, the new proposals were focusing on coverage, leaving patient safety in the dust.

So then the debate raged on, focused entirely on universal health insurance coverage, how much we had to pay for premiums, and whether or not the government should take over the H.M.O. business. While there were some merits to making the insurance industry subject to the anti-trust laws to end 50 years of collusion in price gouging and arbitrary denials, the issues of health insurance have been irrelevant for the reasons as stated multiple times. With so much mayhem, Obama was not doing us any favors with universal coverage. As far as whether we have government or corporate management of health care services, it makes no difference; we're screwed either way.

As for the Republicans, they should stop attacking the only means that victims have for getting a little justice against hospitals, nursing homes, doctors and nurses who continue to regularly commit wanton acts of gross negligence and neglect to the point that it often becomes abusive.

Therefore, the real change we needed was for Congress to take a look at the standard methods of health care delivery and impose some patient safety standards. We needed a special committee to look at hospital mistakes for starters, with experts who could present evidence and call in some hospital administrators for questioning.

Here are a few of the questions that such congressional committee members should ask during the probative hearings:
1. At the time that you set up your nurse-staffing schedule two months in advance and you realized that you would not have enough nurses to provide safe care, what action do you take?
2. Do you notify patients and family members when you have an unsafe nurse staffing level on any given shift?
3. What is the average nurse-to-patient ratio in your intensive care units?
4. What is your average response time to the patient call light?
5. Do your nurses provide fall risk assessment for every new patient?
6. What percentage of your medical equipment is in disrepair?
7. Do your nurses check patients for skin integrity every shift?
8. Do you provide a pressure ulcer risk assessment on every new patient?
9. Do maintain an operating staff on the premises 24 hours per day, 7 days per week for emergency surgery?
10. What is the average waiting time in your emergency department for a patient to see a doctor?
11. Do you monitor compliance with hand washing protocols among your personnel by taking random hand swabs daily?
12. Do you monitor hospital acquired infections and

investigate the source in all cases?
13. Do your nurses turn immobilized patients every two hours without fail and document each position?
14. What steps do your people take to insure against foreign body retention after surgery?
15. What steps do your people take to insure against wrong surgical procedure or operating on the wrong body part?
16. What steps do your management people take to make certain that life-saving equipment is in good working order at all times?
17. What safety measures do you have in place to prevent medication errors?
18. How does your institution deal with polypharmacy issues?

Additionally, the members of the proposed Congressional Committee on Patient Safety in the "United States of Utopia" could access reports filed on the Medicare website to call in the worst offenders in their respective states and who fared the worst with the quality indicators[26]. They could also find out what we need in terms of legislation for patient safety[27].

Finally, Obama and the members of his former rubber stamp Congress needed to get serious about public safety and stop the mass killing and injuring. Making health care safer would substantially have reduced the number of law suits and the higher costs associated with defensive medicine. Therefore, if President Obama had made patient safety his first priority and removed the license to steal from the insurance companies, then maybe he would have accomplished the change we needed. The actions that I speak of are neither left wing nor conservative; it's just common

---

[26] http://medicare.gov
[27] http://www.leapfroggroup.org/

sense to identify an obvious problem and fix it. Unfortunately, in the world of politics, if certain actions don't fit right or left and serve to feed the pigs at the trough, no one will even mention that the problem exists.

The Chains of Change

When the push for health care reform first began in January of 2009, President Barack Obama presented a paragraph about improving patient safety and quality of care in his eight point plan:

"Improve Patient Safety and Quality Care. The plan must ensure the implementation of proven patient safety measures and provide incentives for changes in the delivery system to reduce unnecessary variability in patient care. It must support the widespread use of health information technology and the development of data on the effectiveness of medical interventions to improve the quality of care delivered."

Now, team Obama had a different approach. From a president whose campaign slogan was "The change we need", we should expect changes; however, I never expected him to change his mind about what to change. I thought that somebody had gotten through to him with the reports of so many unnecessary deaths and catastrophic injuries in America hospitals. Obviously he must have seen something on it or he would not have made it part of his "eight step program" for health care reform. What was even more disturbing was that Obama's opponents were not talking about patient safety either. Why does everyone in politics and health care seem to display such depraved indifference to human life and suffering?

In any event, with all of the emphasis on health coverage,

Obama shifted his direction and veered off-course. If he had kept his focus on saving lives by encouraging congress to set patient safety standards, no one could have argued against him without demonstrating a degenerate irreverence to human life. Instead, the left-wing nut jobs in Congress became so emboldened by the White House push for a government-owned HMO that they whipped the single payer system out of the closet and lunged for the brass ring. However, there was such a public outcry against that scheme, that Obama changed the reform focus by dropping the word "care" and replacing it with "insurance" so that he could keep the doctors and hospital owners on board by obliterating patient safety from the rhetoric. Once Obama eliminated concern about the quality of care, he could no longer call it health care reform because he shifted the focus to universal access and who's going to pay for it.

Therefore, since the White had declared open war on the health insurance companies, Republican politicians and conservative media pundits responded by denouncing Democrats as liars.

Barack Obama countered with the following:

"Below are a few points to provide information and suggestions – but the key message to get across is that the lies folks are hearing just aren't true.

"Your letter does not need to include all these points and most importantly should be written in your own words – that's what will make it powerful.

"With premiums growing four times faster than wages, we can't afford not to act. So it's time to set the record straight about special-interest and partisan lies:

"There is no "death panel" mentioned in any of the health reform bills under consideration, and there never

was. Reform only covers optional end-of-life counseling sessions that AARP says protects seniors.

"Reform would stop insurance company rationing of care, not increase it. The bill will be deficit neutral. And numerous fact checkers and the CBO have said the bill would actually strengthen private health insurance.

"The folks spreading these lies are tied to special interests, insurance companies, and partisan attack organizations. Their only goal is to score political points and protect their own profits.

"Reform would:

"make sure insurance companies can't drop your coverage if you get sick or deny you care because you have a pre-existing condition;

"prevent insurers from charging exorbitant co-pays, putting life-time or annual caps on your coverage, or denying you the opportunity to renew your coverage;

"allow young adults to stay on their family coverage until age 26, make it illegal to charge women more for care, and ensure that companies cover preventative care that saves money in the long run."

On the other hand, I am not so sure that the talking points from the "other side" were such big lies. First of all, the so called "death panel" rhetoric came from the proposed requirement for "end-of-life" counseling, which Obama was then saying was "optional". Even as an option, I have been unable to understand how choosing the manner of one's death and having to discuss it with health care providers is going to protect senior citizens.

Second, no one had actually demonstrated that the new health insurance reform law would be "deficit neutral". They haven't published any figures that I could find and they have not told us if they intended to make the delivery of health care more efficient. The Medicare system has been losing 70 billion dollars per year to fraudulent claims according to some estimates; this is the result of contracting the process of examining claims to the private insurance industry. Furthermore, the Medicaid and Medicare systems are more guilty of rationing because they pay doctors and other providers 40-50% less money than the private sector. If that is not rationing, what is?

Third, I don't know who is spreading lies and what lies they are spreading. "Special interests, insurance companies, and partisan attack organizations" seem to be anyone who sees the need for improving health care delivery and coverage but disagrees with President Obama on how to do it. I don't agree with Obama and I am neither a special interest, insurance company nor a partisan attack organization. I happen to be an expert in nursing and patient safety. My father once belonged to a partisan attack organization when he fought against the Nazis during World War II, but I don't think that is what the Obama think tank has in mind.

In conclusion, the next time President Obama wants to put words in our mouths, he should offer us something that won't make us sound like morons.

The Hypocritical Oath of Obama Care

The email circulating from the White House on October 27, 2009 contained a link to twenty videos that people submitted for an advertising campaign. They said that those were the 20 best videos selected from hundreds of entries and that we should vote for the one that they will show repetitively on national television. Well, if those were the best twenty I would really like to see some of the rejects.

Each of the finalist videos was amateurish, corny and stupid. The main theme was that 44 million people die each year due to having no health insurance, so Obama's health insurance reform proposal will save lives. First of all, I would challenge the White House to quote the source of this statistic, because even if you find that among all the people who died in the past year, 44 million did not have health insurance, you cannot conclude that the lack of insurance coverage was the cause of death. On the other hand, if you see that among all the people who died last year, 200,000 died unnecessarily from hospital blunders, you can conclude that our hospitals killed them, while attempting to treat their ailments.

Secondly, the emphasis of all of the White House oratory had switched from quality of care and patient safety to the economic effects of the cost of health insurance premiums. A soon as the AMA made its position clear, the campaign title then shifted from "Health Care Reform" to "Health Insurance Reform." The less publicized fact is that health insurance and health care delivery have merged for the most part into Health Maintenance Organization, Preferred Provider Organizations and other hybrid enterprises design to charge more and provide less. Thus, most health insurance companies own hospitals and physician practices or have managed care contracts that form a partnership with the providers with total control over their financial incentives.

Thirdly, all levels of government own and manage hospitals and clinics and the Feds are operating as owners and insurance carriers with the Veterans Administration, the U.S. public health service, Medicare and Medicaid. Therefore, to attack the insurance industry for inefficiency and denial of care is like the embezzler calling the robber a thief.

Finally, the "Obama Plan" as we found it on the web, spoke of creating outcome incentives, eliminating defensive medicine and appointing doctors and medical experts to identify waste, fraud and abuse. There was nothing about setting basic patient safety standards with funding for enforcement.

Hence, with the long list of benefits of the Obama plan promising, more security and stability, affordable choices, and reining in the cost of health care for all Americans, the Congress has yet to provide us with a law that has even a remote chance of accomplishing any of the above. No one can argue with those advantages but the American people have been vociferously objecting to the thousands of pages of law from left wing-nut politicians who have been running amok. Thus far we have seen frenzied senators and house representatives acting out in the height of their buffoonery; and no one has even attempted to address the clear and present dangers of sloppy and negligent health care causing so much death and injury.

What was the Status Quo?

On December 9, 2009, I got another email from President Obama. It was nice of him to take the time write.

Thomas --

As we head into the final stretch on health reform, big insurance company lobbyists and their partisan allies hope that their relentless attacks and millions of dollars can intimidate us into accepting the status quo.

So I have a message for them, from all of us: Not this time. We have come too far. We will not turn back. We will

not back down.

But do not doubt -- the opponents of reform will not rest. So I need you, the members of **Organizing for America**, to fight alongside me.

We must continue to build out our campaign -- to spread the facts on the air and on the ground, and to bring in more volunteers and train them to join the fight. I urgently need your help to keep Organizing for America's 50-state movement for reform going strong.

Please donate $5 or whatever you can afford today:
https://donate.barackobama.com/FinalStretch
Let's win this together,
President Barack Obama

In response, I'm not sure why he wanted me to give him five dollars. If it was for propaganda to outclass the insurance industry whoopla, both sides were wasting their money because both the HMO people and the politicians are clueless about hospital mistakes, or they know it and don't care. In either case, there was nothing in the proposed legislation about setting standards for patient safety. The Republicans blame the plaintiff malpractice lawyers and the Democrats are lusting for the power and control that socialized medicine with a single payer system has to offer.

Therefore, my answer to President Obama:

"Mr. President, unless and until you and your advisers recognize that the most important component of health care reform must be in setting patient safety standards, so that we can stop the holocaust of hospital victims, I will stay on the sidelines. Start with making it a criminal act to perform a procedure without appropriate training or supervision. Would you permit airlines to place an inexperienced pilot in the cockpit that had to consult the operating manual before take-off?

"You say that the 'other side' wants to maintain the status quo, but you don't really know what the status quo is, so I shall enlighten you. It is the fact that hospitals are the fifth leading cause of death and catastrophic injury in the United States today. That is something that both you and your political opposition seem content to live with. You call for donations and volunteers to 'join the fight'? When you figure out what you're fighting for, then I might jump in for the big win."

Public Option: the Good, the Bad, and the Indifferent

"Public Option" has become a famous (or infamous) buzz word passed down by the Obama propaganda machine; the same one that sent me an email from the President asking me to chip in five bucks for the cause. The reality-check, however, is that no one really knew what "public option" meant. Maybe it was the mystery of it that had everybody so wound up. From all of the bickering and media banter among the talking heads we could see that it meant four different things to four different camps in the great health care debate; the uncovered, the HMO denizens, the Conservative voices of opposition and the star-struck Obama nation dwellers. First, to the "health-coverage challenged", public option looked like a ray of hope until we see that the deal doesn't start until after 2012, if we get past the end of the Mayan calendar. Meanwhile, we get the idea that Uncle Sam was going to be the new doctor in town and doctor knows best. Maybe if we selected the public option we'd all be walking around with our social security number bar codes tattooed on our foreheads so that the medical history can pop-up on the receptionist's computer screen every time we walk into a "public option" medical office. Second, to the HMO customers, public option meant letting everybody else into the waiting room, so it would be impossible to have enough doctors to go around. Additionally, everybody ends up receiving medical treatment for one thing or another with or without coverage. Anyway, Obama promised repeatedly that you can keep what you have, so that question boiled down to whether or not he was a liar. The frightening aspect of public option was the lack of attention to patient safety and the veil of secrecy being thicker in the public sector. To find out what percentage of the 200,000 wrongful death victims per year were patients of government owned hospitals was another matter.

Third, the conservative talking heads didn't like the public option and were worried about who was going to pay to cover the uninsured. The problem with the talking heads was that they talked a lot but didn't have anything to say about the health care industry and what had been going on.

Fourth, the Congressional Democrats, the scariest group of all, were pushing legislation through Congress without reading the bills, which were each more than one thousand pages of gibberish. To them it seemed like the public option was a means to consolidate their fleeting power. They seem to be willing to pass anything as long as it would make most people dependent on Uncle Sam for their health and well-being. Imagine Homeland Security or some other bumbling government agency having access to everyone's medical files.

Consequently, the only thing we can know about the so called "public option" is that in the real world it had absolutely no connection with health care reform. Finally, I never thought anyone would do well with Uncle Sam as the doctor but if one needed to see a proctologist one could make an appointment with the I.R.S.

Health Care Bill: Ploufe!!! Now you see it—now you don't!

On December 23, 2009, David Ploufe, President Barack Obama's chief political strategist sent me an email extolling the virtues of the phantom health care/insurance reform bill. The following was a list of alleged benefits:
1. Extend coverage to 31 million Americans, the largest expansion of coverage since the creation of Medicare;
2. Ensure that you can choose your own doctor;
3. Finally stop insurance companies from denying coverage due to a pre-existing condition;
4. Make sure you will never be charged exorbitant premiums on the basis of your age, health, or gender;
5. Guarantee you will never lose your coverage just because you get sick or injured;
6. Protect you from outrageous out-of-pocket expenditures by establishing lifetime and annual limits;
7. Allow young people to stay on their parents' coverage until they're 26 years old;
8. Create health insurance exchanges, or "one-stop shops" for individuals purchasing insurance, where insurance companies are forced to compete for new customers;
9. Lower premiums for families, according to the non-partisan Congressional Budget Office—especially for struggling folks who will receive subsidies;
10. Help small businesses provide health care coverage to their employees with tax credits and by allowing them to

purchase coverage through the exchanges;
11. Improve and strengthen Medicare by eliminating waste and fraud (without cutting basic benefits), beginning to close the Medicare Part D donut hole, and extending the life of the Medicare trust fund;
12. Create jobs by reining in costs -- fostering competition, reducing waste and inefficiency, and starting to reward doctors and hospitals for quality, not quantity, of care;
13. Cut the deficit by over $130 billion in the next 10 years.

The only thing that had any semblance to an attempt to improve patient safety in hospitals and other institutions is # 12, which says that our doctors and hospitals will get more pay if they don't kill anybody. As long as they keep killing 200,000 people per year, hospital charges and doctors' fees should be real cheap. Maybe that's how they're going to balance the budget. That should give the American public a serious clue that the new health care system is about expanding its role as a killing field.

Wrap Up

Taking a closer look at "health care" we first need to ask, "What is it?" So, we have three major divisions: diagnosis, treatment and assistance with activities of daily living. For the purpose of this discussion, we shall focus on the first two and leave the third as a separate issue, which is mostly about care for the disabled and frail elderly. Additionally, there is a trend leaning toward prevention.

To begin with, diagnosis, which in a conventional sense we can define as attempting to identify the cause of one or more symptoms, does not have the same meaning for all practitioners. Some practitioners focus their attention on only the physical symptoms, others attend only to mental health issues and some take a holistic approach recognizing that all aspects of life can be contributory in causing disease. In any case, we can all agree that diagnostic technology has advanced in the last fifty years to the extent that exploratory surgery has become virtually obsolete. Diagnostic procedures have become considerably less invasive and therefore less risky. Yet there are still more than a few invasive diagnostic procedures that can injure and kill patients, like spinal taps and various endoscopy procedures (inserting a fiber optic scope into a body orifice to view the inside of internal organs). Thus, to have real reform we need patient safety standards for all invasive diagnostic procedures and laws to impose criminal penalties for causing death by failure to abide. For example, we need to look at the method for teaching students and residents, who often perform invasive diagnostic procedures without adequate training and no supervision

To continue, the treatment side of health care is a vast chaotic conundrum of all kinds of modalities emanating from a variety of cultural philosophies and experiences. Of course, every society has its own variation on the theme as evidence by the fact that alternative remedies are more in the mainstream in some countries than others. In our society, we are mostly dominated by a medical autocracy called the American Medical Association, the American Hospital Association and the pharmaceutical industry. Thus the business at hand is cutting, burning, sewing, and chemicals for altering the body's natural responses. We are a society indoctrinated to believe that "Doctor knows best." Although many people survive and become well after being subjected to what health care there is to offer, it is by now common knowledge that there are alternatives to conventional health care that work. Be that as it may, true health care reform has to have a starting point.

Consequently, if we look at the fact that health care is the fifth leading cause of death in the U.S. today, we desperately need to start with patient safety standards in all phases of health care and in all clinical settings. Thus far the medical autocracy has been successful in convincing Obama and Congress to give the health care industry a pass in considering whether practitioners should be held criminally liable for deaths or injuries due to wanton carelessness and callous disregard for the patient's safety and well-being. After Obama's meetings with top industry representatives, he suddenly changed his campaign rhetoric from "Health care reform" to "Health insurance reform."

In conclusion, the answer to the question in the subtitle is that to have any real health care reform we need to start by reducing the risk of having to deal with the reality that health care practitioners in hospitals are killing more people than most of the diseases that caused the victims to seek the care. We can accomplish such a goal by devising a clear set of standards for patient safety, enacting those standards into law and imposing criminal penalties for all whose wanton failure to comply causes survivable injury or death.

12. Health Care "Reform" in 2010

The Crooked Wheel is still the only Game in Town

So there we were one year after the Democrats proposed radical new legislation to change our American health care experience and make it affordable to all. Nothing happened. Obama failed to push his agenda through despite an overwhelming majority in both houses of Congress. By the beginning of 2010 they were back to the drawing board trying to salvage what they could from a failed leadership. The party in power could not sell its new health plan because they did not rally around the most important issue of all—saving lives. At first, patient safety was part of a list of eight reform talking points somewhere near the bottom and then the idea of improving it disappeared altogether from the political horizon. The name of the plan suddenly changed from "Health Care Reform" to "Health Insurance Reform".

Therefore, Obama did not have a rallying point like let's save 200,000 lives per year by setting up patient safety standards in hospitals as we do in the airline industry. What if air travel was the fifth leading cause of death in the United States? Would anyone be crazy enough to buy a ticket? Yet we submit to hospital care whenever we need it without giving safety a second thought. The truth is that an astute leader would have seized the opportunity to address the American public and say, "What are we talking about here? The next person killed by mistake in a hospital could be you or someone you love! So let's do something about it now!" If saving lives had become the major focus rather than saving money, no one could argue against it.

Finally, if the administration could have exercised true leadership they would have encouraged the members of Congress and their respective constituents to focus on creating patient safety standards and simultaneously eliminate the collusive price gouging being perpetrated by insurance companies like Aetna, Vista, Humana and others. It now costs about $182 per person per month for a health care plan with a $10,000 per year deductible. Every time someone goes online for a quote, they are saying, we will take your money while you keep paying for your health care, so that by the time you reach your deductible, you can't afford your premium so we can cancel your policy for non-payment.

The Quality Debate Rages on

After joining the discussion forums on Amazon, I started a thread about health care quality issues and got into a debate with a doctor who called himself "Intrepid." He presented many of the standard arguments that we have been hearing regarding the over-all state of health care delivery in America and that it's the best in the world, even with the casualties. This recap will provide insight as to why the medical establishment continues to refuse to accept responsibility for its failures.

After placing my blog, "What would real health care reform look like?" on the Amazon health care forum, I received an interesting retort arguing that the current state of health care quality is the best we can expect because human error is unavoidable. What follows are my responses to that argument.

Intrepid says: Respectfully, your premise is specious. How much quality assurance and continuous quality improvement ALREADY goes on in every health care institution? How many 3 inch binders of policy and procedure already exist in each hospital?

- One nursing supervisor said hers had literally about 7 feet worth of them in preparation for their Joint Commission on Accreditation of Healthcare Organizations (JCAHO) review."

My response: Quality assurance committees and job functions are ineffective given that the same mistakes keep happening repeatedly in every hospital across the country. That tells us that there are flaws in the basic design and structure of how things are run. There is also no accountability and risk managers have become adept at covering up mistakes so that the patients and family members who survive unscathed never find out that there was a screw up.

Moreover, the JCAHO reviews are a sham. JCAHO notifies the hospital that they are coming three months in advance of inspection. The management puts the hospital staff into over drive to prepare. The inspectors find that the hospital is operating according to patient safety standard. They check everything having to do with patient safety and quality assurance. After the inspectors give the hospital a passing grade and leave, the hospital managers usually throw a big party and life goes back to normal. Therefore, the only assurance we have from the accreditation process is that once every three years the hospital is operating according to standard for three months."

Intrepid says: How many audits go on from managed care, state, Medicaid, Medicare, private insurer, DHS, in addition to hospital utilization review and quality improvement? One time I checked and 9 groups potentially audited one patient's record!"

My response: Third party payers are doing those audits you mention mostly for checking the DRG and ICDM9 billing codes against the charts to make certain that the hospitals are not overcharging them. Their primary interest is saving money; not lives."

Intrepid says: We all want perfection but the person who is doing nursing or physician care is still a human being. Your own children who made mistakes growing up do not transform into superhuman beings free of making unintended mistakes when they go out to do any occupation."

My response: Well of course humans make mistakes; but would you fly commercial airliners that were crashing one plane every week? If that were the case, wouldn't the public rightfully demand that the government step in and establish and enforce improved safety standards? Pilots and other personnel go through a list of redundant safety checks before every flight because mistakes kill people and they know it. The pilots and crew are extra careful because their own lives are also on the line. Furthermore, I am not referring to a few honest mistakes. I am referring to the fact that there are just too many people knowingly violating safety protocols, too many people performing procedures without adequate training and supervision, patients incurring traumatic injuries from falls because no one is meeting their basic needs and the like.

Intrepid says: One study I read too long ago to recall citation said the error rate was about 0.6% in health care overall. Compare that with an average of 160 defects per car in one GM run car assembly plant. How many times would a Morbidity and Mortality or Quality Improvement meeting be held because of even 1 of those 160 defects?"

My response: Automobile defects are a good example of the points I am making here. I am glad you brought it up. Whenever there is a notable defect that causes a few accidents, the press, the government and the public outcry comes down on the manufacturer like a ton of bricks. I cite you two recent infamous episodes: the Ford Bronco blowout epidemic about five years ago and the more recent fiasco with Toyotas causing accidents with accelerators that get stuck. Those problems got eliminated because otherwise the companies and their managers would be held accountable. Congress holds investigative hearings when there is a big issue of public safety. Why have we not had any government intervention with regard to patient safety in hospitals? The reason is that the medical autocracy has been effective in its lobbying and propaganda. The result is that people for the most part have resigned themselves to believing that all the carnage is "unfortunate but unavoidable."

Intrepid says: The bottom line is that humans do health care services. They should try hard to eliminate errors. But it is a principle of practice and a goal not something that can be fully achieved because humans do this work. A lot of extreme effort already is done each day they work to try to create a quality product."

My response: My misguided friend, you are simply not in touch with the reality of hospital life. I don't know what "extreme effort" you are referring to, but when you see two nurses drop an old woman on the floor and put her back to bed without reporting it to anyone and then find the patient with multiple leg fractures after she was screaming in pain for three days, you can hardly call that an "honest mistake". I'm sorry to disillusion you but the reality is that there are too many people in the health industry whose lackluster performance has created unnecessary risk of death and survivable injury just by going for health care services. That is a public safety issue of immense proportions. We can save a great many of those 200,000 people who are dying every year. That is one unnecessary death every 22 minutes."

Intrepid says: "I am not a hospital executive. I am a

physician and I frankly don't care for your 'holier than thou' badgering or accusatory tone. You have made mistakes in your career. Your child if you have one likewise. There are problems but I have to take issue with the skewed view that all the events are preventable or the incidents all as alleged. MANY, many cases are settled but the ones involved feel shafted by the insurance agency that did not want to litigate due to cost. I am sure you know that those persons often steadfastly maintain they were innocent of wrong doing. Cases such as shoulder dystocia in child birth that almost always are settled because until possibly this year, it was virtually impossible to prevent. Each settlement, each case drives up costs. Costs that mean fewer people can afford care. That too is the price. You make it seem like the care in the US is awful. It really is not if you are objective and compare other nations.

"As of 10 years ago, UK care was abysmal in QA compared to the US – by their admission. It was made far better in the past 3 years due to concerted programs to improve care plus incentive programs to reduce errors. Perfection 100% of the time is a goal. We try very hard to achieve that. But it is humanly unattainable. Our costs for health care in the USA are 1/3 to 2/5 higher than other countries due to a litigious attitude that drives up cost far higher than in other nations. The quality of care is not commensurately worse. Even Karl Rove agrees that our litigiousness is in dire need of tort reform. Otherwise care will be increasingly driven to become unaffordable. In private moments we reflect on the implications of law suits on health care costs as well as the psyches of people who were doing their best to serve others.

My response: Okay, so you're a physician. You said you were involved in management and quality assurance. But now I know where you are coming from. You still fail to acknowledge that there is a problem with patient safety in hospitals. You are whining about malpractice insurance premiums, which seems to be your pet peeve and you blame plaintiff lawyers for the onslaught of lawsuits pretending that most cases are frivolous because doctors are wrongfully accused of complications they cannot prevent. Frankly, that is the standard lie. The truth is that plaintiff lawyers have to risk six figures to invest in the cost of malpractice litigation and they are only inclined to do that when there is hard evidence of real negligence, like a patient walking around with sponges or surgical instruments in a body cavity, or someone who underwent somebody else's surgery, while his own condition remained untreated.

Thus now it's clear that to you, real health care reform is to reduce the number of law suits by removing the financial incentive of contingency lawyers. Okay, we can discuss that aspect later but experience has shown that attacking the lawyers' income structures doesn't work. Victims continue to seek justice and lawyers have demonstrated that they will work for less to fill the need. In addition, at least one of those fee reducing state laws have already been struck down as unconstitutional in Federal Court.

But first, let me clarify some things because for you there are only absolutes. If I say we need for Congress to impose patient safety standards and make those who are grossly negligent and guilty of dereliction of duty owed to patients criminally liable for causing death or survivable injury, you respond by saying, 'nobody's perfect.' If I point out that health care is itself the fifth leading cause of death in the United States, you respond by saying that care in the U.S. is not as awful as I make it seem. Those are not valid arguments. If you want to challenge the facts, do so, because your obvious defensive posturing is proving my point; the failure of the medical community to acknowledge that hospital care is flawed in its design like a bridge that is destined to collapse or an accident that is waiting to happen.

To continue, Medicare has thus far identified 28 "never events" for which it and all other third party payers refuse reimburse hospitals. These are adverse events that should never happen, like failure to exercise reasonable precaution to prevent traumatic injuries from falling, stage IV bedsores, etc. Such events have become pandemic and hospitals have built in hazards. There is an identifiable risk to simply entering a hospital for admission, even if a majority of patients have good outcomes and adverse events like unexpected drug reactions that can't be prevented. If you deny the truth rather than becoming part of the solution, you become part of the problem."

How Affordable is the Affordable Care Act?

The new Patient Protection and Affordable Care Act of 2010 is a sham. It looks like there is going to be more access to health care plans at lower cost, but it's a mirage. First of all, the table of contents in the 974-page law document is all screwed up so it will take all day to find any particular section. There are also a myriad of confusing amendments and add-ons that have nothing to do with the so-called health insurance changes so there is a huge hurdle in trying to understand this new statute. Enforcing this law is going to be virtually impossible because each of the insurance companies will have a team of lawyers with legal opinions that their company's practices are compliant with the new law. Since nobody can understand it anyway, there will be no one to challenge them.

Secondly, for pre-existing condition coverage we have to

pay a $2,500 per year deductible and 20% of all health fees and charges until we have spent $6,000 out of pocket while paying premiums every month. Where is the change? That is exactly what is available now for an individual buying a plan directly from an insurance company who is 55 to 64 years of age with a few minor medical problems under control like arthritis, diabetes or hypertension. The only difference is that starting in 2014; insurance companies won't be allowed to turn anyone down for pre-existing conditions. But you will still have to eat the deductible and co-pay totaling $6,000 per year and pay extra for being in the high risk pool.

Thirdly, if you have no pre-existing condition and you can't afford full coverage you will have to take a plan with a high deductible from $1,500 to $10,000. Since the average healthy person spends less than $1,500 per year on doctor's visits, you will be paying premiums for nothing because you will have to pay full price for doctors' visits. So, nothing has changed for those who can't afford the cost of low or no deductibles.

Fourthly, if you have no insurance and need health care now the new website http://healthcare.gov refers you to an existing family health care center or facility obligated by the Hill-Burton Act to provide care to indigent people. If you need care urgently you will have to wait about one month for a specialist appointment in most cases. This waiting time will not change under the new law, so the promise of quicker access of the uninsured poor to health care was a lie.

Finally, the patient protection aspect of this new law is a joke. The new statute creates a hodgepodge of new federally funded research programs to find ways to improve quality. There is not one section on establishing standards of patient safety; it only makes the pork barrel deeper and wider for the politicians and their cronies to feed their greed.

In conclusion, the new health care law is a bogus shell game. The underinsured will remain as such with the high deductibles still in place. The people with pre-existing conditions will be subjected to high deductibles so they will have to pay out of pocket for most services related to those conditions in addition to the premiums. Access to healthcare for the poor uninsured who are not eligible for Medicaid will remain the same; waiting more than one month for an appointment to see a specialist.

Patient Protection and Affordable Care: The Fool's Paradise

On March 23, 2010, Barak Obama signed the Patient Protection and Affordable Care bill into law. Now we have to ask the question, "Do we really have patient protection and affordable care?" Where is it? When I reviewed the new law I couldn't find any patient protection; and the term "affordable" begs the question, "Affordable by whom?" Health care is affordable to people like President Obama, Bill Gates, George Soros and Michael Bloomberg. But for the rest of us, why would any thinking person believe that a $6,000 per year out of pocket cost over premiums is "affordable?" That's more than what most people spend for health care in the real world, so that most of us are paying health care premiums for nothing. Furthermore, if you want zero deductible you have to pay about $7,200, which is five times more than what the average person pays privately for health care per year. Hence the price we pay is solely for financial protection against the cost of catastrophic illness or injury.

Universal Coverage

The reality is that there is still no universal coverage and there is no provision for it in the new law. There is only "near-universal coverage. Section 1501 (2) (D) states, "The requirement achieves near-universal coverage by building upon and strengthening the private employer-based health insurance system, which covers 176,000,000 Americans nationwide." This tells us that the 45 million working poor and some 25 million illegal aliens will have to continue using the emergency rooms for primary care.

The U.S. government will continue to spend about $600 per visit to treat non-emergencies via the Hill-Burton Act instead of $60 for a walk-in clinic visit. Thus, this new act of Congress changes nothing. Moreover, the new act is not intended to provide universal coverage. That idea was lobbed off in the back rooms of the Congressional building. SEC.10106. AMENDMENTS TO SUBTITLE F amends Section 1501 (a) (2) (E) reads as follows:

"The economy loses up to $207,000,000,000 a year because of the poorer health and shorter lifespan of the uninsured. By significantly reducing the number of the uninsured, the requirement, together with the other provisions of this Act, will significantly reduce this economic cost."

Therefore, we can conclude that Congress merely intended to reduce the number of uninsured persons without specifying the goal in numbers, how to accomplish it and by when. The people who currently have medical coverage are: 1) those whose employers provide health plans; 2) people who are Medicaid eligible who are able to fill out forms and sit in government offices; 3) those who are over 65 years of age or disabled, thus qualifying for Medicare 4) Self-employed wealthy private purchasers. The people who don't have coverage are the rest of the population who simply cannot afford to pay $10,000 per year for health care, including the homeless and those with diminished mental capacity who are otherwise eligible for Medicaid. The Congressional answer to this dilemma is a demonstration project to provide access to comprehensive coverage to the uninsured at "reduced rates" in 10 States giving full discretion to the Secretary of Health and Human Services as to the logistics.

Cost Savings Focus on Preventive Care

Section 2713 provides for coverage of preventive health services. The statue requires coverage for all recommendations classified as "A" or "B" by the United States Preventive Services Task Force. This is redundant since all of those recommendations such as routine screenings for prevalent diseases in pregnant women, newborn infants, young children, and adult males and females are already available as standard services in virtually all health care settings. The problem is that the uninsured have no access to such prevention services and are therefore much more likely to sicken unnecessarily and die prematurely.

In conclusion, there are no additional cost savings benefits from this new law. Furthermore, as the number of undocumented illegal aliens continues to grow with more insurance premiums subject to free market enterprise with no anti-gouging regulations, the number of uninsured and underinsured will continue to grow with an increase in premature mortality.

Lip Service on Duplication of Services

Mr. Jones goes to his primary care physician (PCP) with a

complaint of left flank pain and blood in his urine. The doctor suspects kidney stones and sends the patient to the lab for a series of blood and urine tests that include screening for kidney function and urinary tract infection. Thus far, this is the prudent way to practice medicine as the doctor must have a base line for electrolytes, blood count, urinalysis and screen for abnormalities. The lab receives $385.00 from the third party payer. The patient also goes to a radiology center for a sonogram and X-rays for a cost of $1,850.00, the total being $2,235.00. Following this initial work up, the PCP refers Mr. Jones to an urologist to confirm the primary diagnosis and recommend a treatment plan.

The specialist has one policy; all new patients must have complete blood work, urinalysis, x-rays and sonography. It doesn't matter that the urologist has access to all of the results from tests done a few days prior to the visit even if the patient goes back to the same lab and radiology center. The patient must go for a complete identical set of tests for another cost of $2,235.00. Multiply this duplication by tens of millions and we have an annual waste of over a billion dollars. One would think that the new law could easily put a stop to this blatant abuse. Whether the motivation is profiteering or defensive medicine makes no difference; the physicians are the ones who order the tests so they have complete control. Since this phenomenon continues unabated, we need some form of legislation to modify physician behavior.

The insurance companies can refuse to pay for the duplication, but then the financial liability shifts to the patient who will have to suffer harassment at the hands of unscrupulous collection agencies, as well as being dragged into court. One would think that the new law would have some provision that would penalize any doctor who ordered a duplication of diagnostic tests that were done within a specified number of days of the original results. However, such is not the case. There is only vague lip service as follows:

"SEC. 3502: ESTABLISHING COMMUNITY HEALTH TEAMS TO SUPPORT THE PATIENT-CENTERED MEDICAL HOME: (G) promote effective strategies for treatment planning, monitoring health outcomes and resource use, sharing information, treatment decision support, and organizing care to avoid duplication of service and other medical management approaches intended to improve quality and value of health care services."

Therefore, since there is nothing in the new law that expressly prohibits doctors from ordering duplicate diagnostic tests, this behavior will continue unabated, draining billions of dollars from the economy with the excess costs being passed on to the consumers.

Wrap Up

As the year of 2010 came to a close, it became clear that the idea of real health care reform was nothing more than a red herring. The Patient Protection and Affordable Health Care Act is a testimonial to the greatest sellout in history. The title of the law is by itself a lie because no one is going to protect the patients and health care will never become affordable with high deductibles plus premiums. The bottom line is that with all of that one-sided political power, Obama couldn't sell his radical health care reform plan because even many of his Congressional cronies listened to the public outrage and shied away from the socialist reforms called "the public option."

Consequently, the Obama strategists had to initiate plan "B"—eliminate the public option, drop the patient safety issues, leave about 31 million people sucking wind, let the private HMO's gouge the public for another four years before they cut and run and get out the phony dog-and-pony show to promote imaginary preventive health measures for the planet No-go; to magically turn all of the inner-city rat holes into environment-friendly homes with purified air and plenty of sunshine. Of course, after the carnage, Obama or his successor will walk among the smoldering rubble, dead bodies and the dying and say, "You see, we told you that the 'public option' was the only way to go!"

13. FDA = Fraud, Deception and Abuse

One of the greatest dangers we have ever faced as a nation is the transformation of our society into a drug culture. We have pills available for every feeling of discomfort; pain, anxiety, rage, depression, anguish and hyperactivity to name a few and pills to control every body function like heart rate, blood sugar, blood pressure, urine flow, digestion, defecation, hormone secretion, reproduction, neurological function, heart rate and the like. It's as if we are not supposed to feel anything or take responsibility for healthy diet with natural supplements and exercise.

Pharmaceutical companies manufacture thousands of different types of designer drugs in an industry that is raking in hundreds of billions of dollars per year. Consequently, the Food and Drug Administration (FDA) is our only safety net with regard to our food supply and the drugs and medical devices that our doctors prescribe. Tainted food products have the capacity to spread fatal disease and every medication has a potential for side effects that cause catastrophic injury or death. The idea behind this level of protection is to safeguard the integrity of the food to prevent contamination and require medical product manufacturers to tell us the actual risks and accurately report the intended therapeutic effect, so that we can decide if the benefit we seek is worth gambling with our lives. However, if the information is unreliable or false, then the game is fixed and any bet is a guaranteed loss.

Regarding medical issues, the underlying disease is often so devastating that patients will take the chance; but they are all relying on the FDA to keep the pharmaceutical and medical device manufacturers in line. Most of us believed for decades that the criteria for new drug and contrivance approval was stringent enough to be able trust the manufacturer's label. Now we know that the system has been totally corrupt with bribery and extortion. What's even worse is that what should have been the scandal of the millennium virtually escaped public attention through a massive cover-up scheme that involved the mainstream media looking the other way. Perhaps the truth was too horrible for anyone to face or for any elected or selected official to accept responsibility for it; but the truth must nonetheless be told and we, the public, must wake up to the reality that the chaos of tainted food and toxic pharmaceuticals putting us in harm's way is already upon us.

The FDA Approval Process: Bribery, Coercion and Extortion

Before January of 2009, it was clear that the practice of a manufacturer funding its clinical trial was a model that was biased in favor of corporate profits and therefore not ideal. However, it turned out to be much worse. Now that we have rediscovered that the FDA has been a cesspool of corruption with officials taking bribes to approve drugs that have not been adequately tested, how can we trust any prescription or the doctors who write them?

Moreover, corrupt FDA decision makers who pass approvals without requiring standard verifications along with the dirt-bags who pay the bribes to sell their "miracle-cure" poisons, falsifying clinical trial reports, are mass murderers, with a depraved indifference to human life; the same as all of the illicit drug lords and their gang members. Now, there is proof that was buried by the media and never spoken of publicly in Congress. So let us review this evidence and then follow the trail to see what action if any that Obama and his Congress took.

First, we have a certificate of authentication from Frederick J. Saddler, Director of Freedom of Information of the Department of Health and Human Services, as shown here.

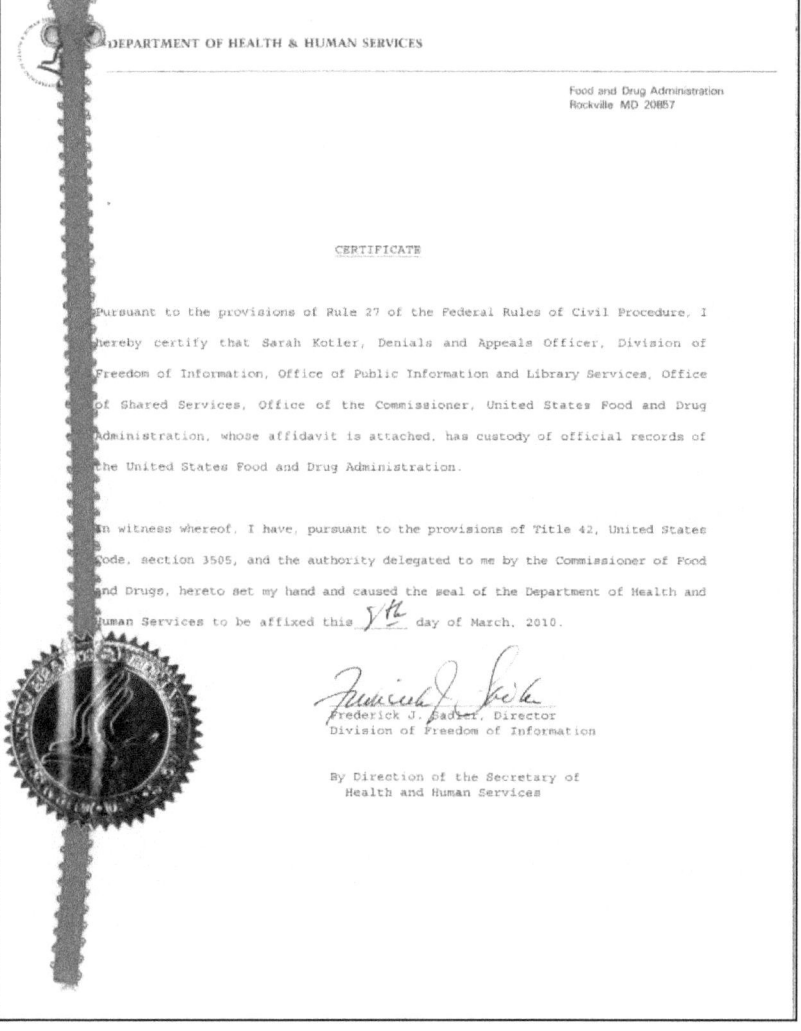

Second, we have a copy of sworn affidavit from Sarah Kotler who was the Denials and Appeals Officer of the Division of Freedom of Information, Office of Public Information and Library Services, Office of Shared Services, Office of the Commissioner, United States Food and Drug Administration who authenticated the documentation of corruption as shown here.

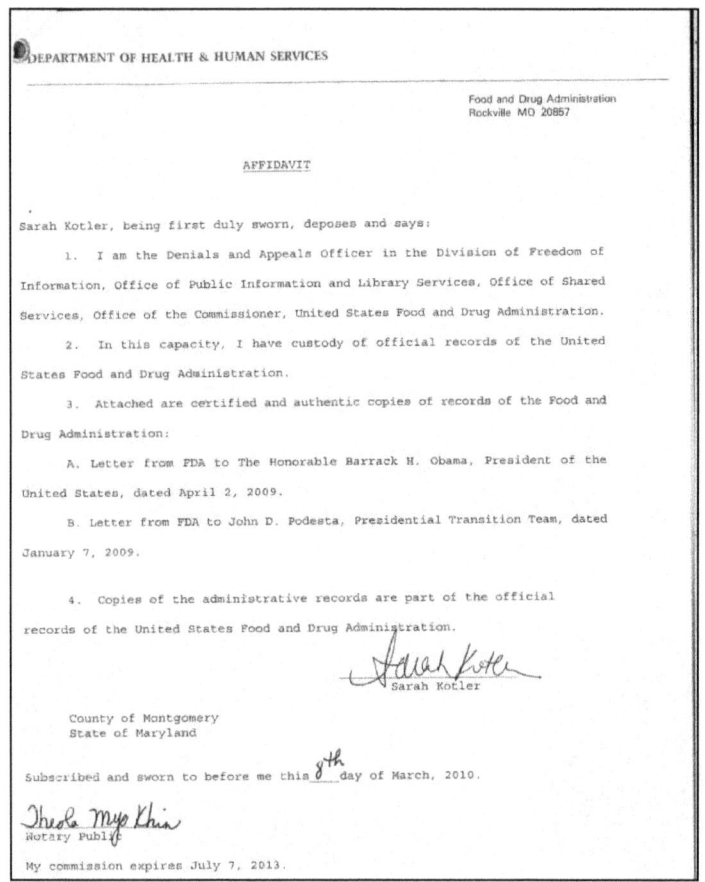

Third, we have a letter to John D. Podesta, head of the Presidential Transition Team, dated January 9, 2009 from certain whistle blowers, with the signatures redacted.

"Dear Mr. Podesta:

"We, physicians and scientists of the U.S. Food and Drug Administration (FDA), fully support the agenda of President Obama to 'challenge the status quo in Washington and to bring about the kind of change America needs.' America urgently needs change at FDA because FDA is fundamentally broken, failing to fulfill its mission, and because re-establishing a proper and effectively functioning FDA is vital to the physical and economic health of the nation. As stated in the November 2007 FDA Science Board Report entitled *FDA Science and Mission at Risk;* 'A strong FDA is crucial for the health of our country. The benefits of a robust, progressive Agency are enormous; the risks of a debilitated, under-performing organization are incalculable. The FDA constitutes a critical component of our nation's healthcare delivery and public health system. The FDA, as much as any public or private sector institution in our country, touches the lives, health and well-being of all Americans. . . . The FDA is also central to the economic health of the nation, regulating approximately $1 trillion in consumer products or 25 cents of every consumer dollar expended in this country annually. . . . The importance of the FDA in the nation's security is similarly profound. . . . Thus, the nation is at risk if FDA science is at risk.'

"The purpose of this letter is to inform you that the scientific review process for medical devices at FDA has been corrupted and distorted by current FDA managers, thereby placing the American people at risk. Through this letter and your action, we hope that future FDA employees will not experience the same frustration and anxiety that we have experienced for more than a year at the hands of FDA managers because we are committed to public integrity and were willing to speak out. Currently, there is an atmosphere at FDA in which the honest employee fears the dishonest employee, and not the other way around. Disturbingly, the atmosphere does not yet exist at FDA where honest employees committed to integrity and the FDA mission can act without fear of reprisal. This letter provides an inside view of the severely broken science, regulation and administration at the Center for Devices and Radiological Health (CDRH) that recently forced FDA physicians and scientists to seek direct intervention from the U.S. Congress. This letter also provides elements of reform that are necessary to begin real change at FDA from the 'bottom up.'

"Since May 2008, the FDA Commissioner has been provided with irrefutable evidence that managers at CDRH have placed the nation at risk by corrupting and distorting the scientific evaluation of medical devices, and by interfering with our responsibility to ensure the safety and effectiveness of medical devices before they are used on the American public. Before a medical device can be cleared or approved by FDA, the law requires that safety and effectiveness is determined based on 'valid scientific evidence . . . .from which it can fairly and responsibly be concluded by qualified experts that there is reasonable assurance of the safety and effectiveness of the device.' Managers at CDRH have ignored the law and ordered physicians and scientists to assess medical devices employing unsound evaluation methods, and to accept non-scientific, nor clinically validated, safety and effectiveness evidence and conclusions, as the basis of device clearance and approval. Managers with incompatible, discordant, and irrelevant scientific and clinical expertise in devices for which they have the full authority to make final regulatory decisions, have ignored serious safety and effectiveness concerns of FDA experts. Managers have ordered, intimidated, and coerced FDA experts to modify scientific evaluations, conclusions and recommendations in violation of the laws, rules and regulations and to accept clinical and technical data that is not scientifically valid nor obtained in accordance with legal requirements, such as obtaining proper informed consent from human subjects. These same managers have knowingly tried to avoid transparency and accountability by failing to properly document the basis of their non-scientific decisions in administrative records. As examples of wrongdoing, the Director of the Office of Device Evaluation (ODE) has gone so far as to:

- Order physicians and scientists to ignore FDA Guidance documents;
- Knowingly allow her subordinates to issue written threats of disciplinary action if physicians and scientists failed to change their scientific opinions and recommendations to conform to those of management;
- Issue illegal internal documents that do not conform to the requirements of Good Guidance Practices, are not publicly available, and, if followed, would circumvent science and legal regulatory requirements;
- Fail to properly document significant decisions in the administrative files;
- Make, and allow, false statements in FDA documents;
- Allow manufacturers to market devices that have never been approved by FDA;
- Remove Black Box warnings recommended by FDA experts;
- Bypass FDA experts and fail to properly label devices;
- Exclude FDA experts from participating in Panel Meetings because manufacturers 'expressed concerns that [FDA experts] are biased.'

"For seven months, Dr. von Eschenbach and his

Assistant Commissioner for Accountability and Integrity (Mr. Bill McConagha) have conducted a sham investigation resulting in absolutely nothing: no one was held accountable, no appropriate or effective actions have been taken, and the same managers who engaged in the wrongdoing remain in place and have been rewarded and promoted. Dr. von Eschenbach and Mr. McConagha failed to take appropriate or effective actions while the physicians and scientists who had the courage and patriotism to speak out, and who refused to comply with FDA management wrongdoing, have suffered severe and ongoing retaliation. The failure of Dr. von Eschenbach and Mr. McConagha to take appropriate or effective actions has made them complicit in the wrongdoing, has harmed the reputations and lives of individual employees, and has unnecessarily placed the American public at risk.

"In October 2008, the U.S. Congress was provided with the same evidence of wrongdoing that was given to the Commissioner. After Congress examined the evidence, the U.S. House of Representatives Committee on Energy and Commerce sent a letter to the FDA Commissioner dated November 17, 2008, 11 stating that they had 'received compelling evidence of serious wrongdoing . . . and well-documented allegations . . . from a large group of scientists and physicians . . . who report misconduct within CDRH that represents an unwarranted risk to public health and a silent danger that may only be recognized after many years . . . and that physicians and scientists within CDRH who objected [to the misconduct] . . . have been subject to reprisals.'

"Unfortunately, the preceding facts are only the latest examples of shocking managerial corruption, wrongdoing and retaliation at CDRH. Back in February 2002, a biomedical engineer at CDRH reported serious managerial misconduct to the current Director of ODE and ultimately filed an EEOC lawsuit in September 2004. After six long stressful years of hardship and litigation, a Judge issued a forty-two page *Decision and Findings of Fact* concluding that: 'the Agency promoted a hostile working environment . . . permeated with derogatory comments and adverse employment actions . . . the Agency 'failed to exercise any reasonable care to prevent and correct promptly the harassing behavior' . . . the actions toward the engineer were 'unconscionable' and 'occurred openly within the FDA, unchecked, for over four years' . . . that 'FDA managers were aware and failed to take appropriate or effective corrective actions; but rather, demonstrated a systemic disregard for federal regulations as well as the FDA's own policies.' The Judge further concluded: 'supervisors [including the current Director of ODE] knew or should have known of the hostile work environment, but neither the supervisors nor the Agency did anything to correct the situation or prevent further discrimination' . . . and 'failed to exercise any reasonable care to prevent or correct the hostility of [managers] towards the Complainant.' Shockingly, the current Director of ODE herself testified in court that she was aware of the 'hostile work environment' but 'did not want to get involved,' thereby corroborating her complicity in the corruption and retaliation against this employee. These independent facts confirm the longstanding pandemic corruption that cries out for new leadership at FDA from the bottom up.

"We are confident that new leadership from the bottom up will be a top priority of Mr. Daschle as the new Secretary of the Department of Health and Human Services (HHS). As Mr. Daschle has recognized, the integrity of the FDA scientific review and decision-making process, where scientific experts make evaluations and recommendations, must be evidence-based and independent, insulated from improper influences. As a matter of fact, Mr. Daschle points to the 1998 FDA approval of mammography computer-aided detection (CAD) devices as an example of a breakdown of the independent scientific review and decision-making process. These CAD devices were supposed to improve breast cancer detection on mammograms. As Mr. Daschle recognized, post-approval scientific publications revealed that actual clinical performance of these CAD devices did not improve breast cancer detections and they were associated with increased patient recalls and unnecessary breast biopsies. We note that the Agency knowingly approved these devices in 1998 even though there was no clinical evidence of improved cancer detection and, furthermore, the device was never tested in accordance with its intended use—one of the principal required elements for device approval.

"Astoundingly, the approval was based on pseudo-science that consisted of unsubstantiated estimates of potential benefit using flawed testing. Use of these devices is a major public health issue as approximately 40 million mammograms are performed every year in the U.S. Furthermore, as a failure of FDA post approval monitoring, the FDA never carried out any post-marketing assessment or re-evaluation of the clinical performance of these devices, ignoring accumulating clinical evidence provided by independent research publications revealing that these devices were ineffective and potentially harmful when used in clinical practice.

"FDA managers continue to fail to apply even the most fundamental scientific and legal requirements for the approval of these, and so many other, devices. These failures constitute a clear and silent danger to the American public. Since 2006, FDA physicians and scientists have recommended five times not to approve mammography CAD devices without valid scientific and clinical evidence of safety and effectiveness. Manufacturers of these devices have repeatedly failed to provide valid scientific and clinical evidence demonstrating safety and effectiveness of these devices in accordance with the intended use as required by the law. These matters were the subject of a Radiological Devices Panel meeting in March 2008 at which independent outside experts ratified all of the scientific, clinical, and regulatory points of the FDA experts required for proper assessment of the safety and effectiveness of these devices. Despite this, in April of 2008, the Director of ODE ignored the recommendations of all of the experts and approved these devices without any scientific, clinical or legal justification.

"Although unknown to Mr. Daschle and the American public, the Director of ODE and her subordinates committed the most outrageous misconduct by ordering, coercing, and intimidating FDA physicians and scientists to recommend approval, and then retaliating when the physicians and scientists refused to go along. This, and similar management actions with other devices, compelled us to write the FDA Commissioner in May 2008 and, because he utterly failed to take appropriate or effective actions, we later informed the U.S. Congress in October 2008.

"We, physicians and scientists at FDA, seek your immediate attention for change and reform at FDA. To bring real change and reform to FDA, it is absolutely necessary that Congress pass, and the President sign, new legislation providing the strongest possible protections for all government employees, especially physicians and scientists, who speak out about wrongdoing and corruption that interferes with their mission and responsibility to the American public. We desperately need honesty without fear of retaliation for our evaluations and recommendations on medical devices, as well as accountability and transparency, to become the law and thus the foundation of the FDA mission and workplace. We totally agree with the following statement of President Obama: 'Often the best source of information about waste, fraud, and abuse in government is an existing government employee committed to public integrity and willing to speak out. Such acts of courage and patriotism, which can sometimes save lives and often save taxpayer dollars, should be encouraged rather than stifled. We need to empower federal employees as watchdogs of wrongdoing and partners in performance. Barack Obama will strengthen whistleblower laws to protect federal workers who expose waste, fraud, and abuse of authority in government. Obama will ensure that ... whistleblowers have full access to courts and due process.'

"As President Obama has emphasized, he intends to govern the nation and to bring about change from the bottom up. We believe that, as applied to FDA, this means a complete restructuring of the evaluation and approval process such that it is driven by science and carried out by clinical and scientific experts in their corresponding areas of expertise who are charged with review of regulatory submissions in accordance with the laws, rules and regulations. It is necessary that FDA expert physicians and scientists approve final regulatory determinations of safety and effectiveness, rather than multiple layers of managers who are not qualified experts and who often ignore scientific evidence and the law. President Obama has also emphasized the need for complete transparency in government. His Transparency Policy should be mandatory for all FDA regulatory decisions and associated documentation. The longstanding FDA practice of secret meetings and secret communications between FDA managers and regulated industry must be strictly prohibited. Complete transparency in the regulatory decision-making process would serve as a deterrent to wrongdoing and an incentive for excellence.

"FDA also requires major renovation of the organizational structure of the various Centers and Offices to restore internal checks and balances that proactively prevent corruption and manipulation of facts, science, and data. At present, FDA is plagued by a heavy-layered top–down organizational structure that concentrates far too much power in isolated Offices run by entrenched managers where cronyism is paramount. We recommend that the Office of Device Evaluation be dismantled and split into multiple Offices, each headed by a physician or scientist with strong leadership credentials and extensive clinical and technical expertise in the specific devices they regulate. These leadership positions should be rotated on a regular basis. Furthermore, the current system of employee performance evaluation must be eliminated because it is used as an instrument of extortion by management and to terrorize employees who would otherwise serve as 'watchdogs of wrongdoing and partners in performance.' The performance of FDA physicians and scientists must be based on an independent peer review process where extramural experts review the quality of the scientific content of their regulatory work.

"We strongly support the sentiments expressed in a recent letter from Congressman Bart Stupale's complete change in FDA's current leadership. At CDRH, such change can be implemented immediately by removing and punishing all managers who have participated in, fostered or tolerated the well-documented corruption and wrongdoing. All improper management actions, including improper adverse personnel actions, and clearance/approval of medical devices that were not made in accordance with the laws, rules and regulations, must be reversed. Such swift and decisive action of transparency and accountability will send a strong message FDA-wide that wrongdoing will no longer be tolerated. In order to have a truly fresh start, we recommend that the new Commissioner request resignations from management positions by all current managers within CDRH, and use a competitive merit-based process to re-fill AI management positions.

"The FDA mission is not limited to pre-market evaluation of safety and effectiveness. FDA is also responsible for the total product life cycle including actual clinical performance. FDA must not engage in a fire-fighting regulatory posture after medical products are introduced into clinical practice and used on patients. FDA must pursue a culture of proactive regulatory science and remain vigilant in monitoring clinical performance of devices. For FDA to fully accomplish its post-marketing responsibilities there must be complete coordination between FDA and all HHS health-related agencies and institutes. This will provide FDA with the necessary critical scientific capability and capacity to achieve its post-marketing oversight. In turn, FDA will be able to provide the American public and all health care decision makers with objective and scientifically rigorous assessments that synthesize available evidence on diagnosis, treatment and prevention of disease. Ultimately, this will result in a lower health care burden on our society.

"In a time of transition, with the country facing an economic crisis with potential devastating consequences to the American people, we strongly believe that change and reform at

FDA must be a top priority because FDA is central to the physical and economic health of the nation and because it can play a central role in reducing the future healthcare burden and avoiding public health catastrophes. We sincerely hope that, together, we can establish a culture of science, honesty, transparency and integrity at FDA to serve as the genesis of reform for the entire American health care system."

Fourth, we have a letter to President Obama dated April 9, 2009 from certain whistleblowers with the signatures redacted attesting to fraud and corruption on a massive scale, which has plagued the FDA for decades. This letter is a testimonial to the fact that even after the shocking and scandalous revelations presented to the lead dog of the Obama transition team, there was no action, and aside from the resignations of the former commissioner and two of his deputies, the same criminals were are still in charge of the FDA for more than two years after Obama took office.

"Dear Mr. President:

"The purpose of this letter is to draw your attention to the frustration and outrage that FDA physicians and scientists, public advocacy groups, the press, and the American people, have repeatedly expressed over the misdeeds of FDA officials. Recent press reports revealed extensive evidence of serious wrongdoing by Dr. Andrew von Eschenbach, Dr. Frank M. Torti, top FDA attorneys, Center and Office Directors, and many others in prominent positions of authority at FDA. As a result, Dr. Frank M. Torti, Acting Commissioner and the FDA's first Chief Scientist, abruptly left the Agency. But, the many other FDA managers who have failed to protect the American public, who have violated laws, rules, and regulations, who have suppressed or altered scientific or technological findings and conclusions, who have abused their power and authority, and who have engaged in illegal retaliation against those who speak out, have not been held accountable and remain in place.

"On Monday, March 30, 2009, Dr. Joshua Sharfstein, newly appointed Principal Deputy Commissioner, assumed the position of Acting Commissioner until Dr. Margaret Hamburg is confirmed. Numerous FDA physicians and scientists are certain that Dr. Hamburg and Dr. Sharfstein will bring the necessary change to FDA to guarantee integrity, accountability, and transparency, to ensure that all future decisions are solely based on science and in accordance with the laws, rules, and regulations. However, sweeping measures are needed to end the systemic corruption and wrongdoing that permeates all levels of FDA and has plagued the Agency far too long.

The latest example of wrongdoing was reported on March 23, 2009 from a Federal District Court Judge who ruled that FDA's decision on the Plan B drug was 'arbitrary and capricious because they were not the result of reasoned and good faith agency decision-making.' FDA's top leaders at the Center for Drug Evaluation and Research (CDER) testified that they 'didn't have a choice, and . . . [weren't] sure that [they] would be allowed to remain [in their positions if they] didn't agree' to ignore the science and the law. To the contrary, they should be removed from their positions of authority precisely because they didn't follow the science and the law. The judge further ruled that there was 'un-rebutted evidence that the FDA's [decision] stemmed from political pressure rather than permissible health and safety concerns.' The 'improper political influence' and the many 'departures from its own policies' reveal that such FDA officials are incapable of ensuring integrity and science at FDA.

"On October 14, 2008, FDA physicians and scientists

wrote to members of the House Energy and Commerce Committee reporting that top FDA officials at the Center for Devices and Radiological Health (CDRH) had distorted the scientific review of medical devices and then retaliated against those who brought this to light. Two Congressman John Dingell (then Chairman) and Congressman Bart Stupak (Chairman, Subcommittee on Oversight and Investigations) wrote to then FDA Commissioner Dr. Andrew C. von Eschenbach (since resigned), stating that there were 'well-documented allegations that senior managers within CDRH' had acted in violation of the law ... [and that] sweeping measures may be necessary to address the distortion of science alleged by so many CDRH scientists.

"On January 7, 2009, FDA physicians and scientists wrote to Mr. John Podesta: 'Through this letter and your action, we hope that future FDA employees will not experience the same frustration and anxiety that we have experienced for more than a year at the hands of FDA managers because we are committed to public integrity and were willing to speak out. Currently, there is an atmosphere at FDA in which the honest employee fears the dishonest employee, and not the other way around. Disturbingly, the atmosphere does not yet exist at FDA where honest employees committed to integrity and the FDA mission can act without fear of reprisal. ... America urgently needs change at FDA because FDA is fundamentally broken, failing to fulfill its mission, and because reestablishing a proper and effectively functioning FDA is vital to the physical and economic health of the nation.'

"On January 13, 2009, the NY Times reported that FDA officials allowed 'improper political influence' to guide official FDA actions. The Director of the Office of Device Evaluation, Dr. Donna-Bea Tillman, approved a medical device used for the detection of breast cancer despite the fact that all of the FDA experts involved recommended against approval of the device three times. Dr. Tillman's decision to overrule the FDA experts 'followed a phone call from a Connecticut congressman [Christopher Shays].'

"On January 26, 2009, FDA physicians and scientists wrote to you directly seeking your help and recommending that 'you remove and hold accountable all managers who have ordered, participated in, fostered or tolerated the well-documented corruption, wrongdoing and retaliation at the Agency.' That letter was prompted by concerns that FDA officials were planning to investigate physicians and scientists in retaliation for the January 13, 2009 story in the NY Times. These concerns were well founded.

"On March 13, 2009, one week after another episode detailing wrongdoing and improper political influence involving top FDA officials was published in the Wall Street Journal, Acting Commissioner Dr. Frank M. Torti and FDA attorneys sprang into action. Their solution— send an FDA-wide email admonishing FDA employees that they 'must comply with obligations to keep certain information confidential [including] e-mail to and from employees within FDA [that document the] deliberative process' and threatening that 'violation can result in disciplinary sanctions and/or individual criminal liability.'

"These threats did not escape the scrutiny of Senator Chuck Grassley, Ranking Member of the U.S. Senate Committee on Finance. In a letter to Dr. Torti on March 24, 2009, Senator Grassley wrote: 'Your memorandum appears to run contrary to many statutes protecting executive branch communications with members of Congress. I am concerned with the timing of your memorandum, given some recent high profile matters concerning your Agency and the release of information that has shown failures in FDA's regulatory mission. [This] could be viewed as an effort to chill and/or prevent FDA employees from exercising their rights under whistleblower protection laws. Whistleblowers are some of the most patriotic people I know—men and women who labor, often anonymously, to let Congress and the American people know when the Government isn't working so we can fix it.'

"The Wall Street Journal and FDA documents revealed efforts by top FDA officials (including Dr. von Eschenbach, Dr. Torti, Mr. William McConagha, and other FDA attorneys) to cover-up their attempts to improperly influence, obstruct, impede and distort the due and proper administration of the FDA scientific regulatory process involving a knee implant device. According to the Columbia University Journalism Review, 'the [Wall Street] Journal describes a process in this case that's, well, corrupt. I don't know what else you'd call it. It even has a smoking gun.' An advisory committee of outside experts, convened to provide advice on the safety and effectiveness of the knee implant, was misled and manipulated by Dr. Daniel Schultz (Director of CDRH) as well as top FDA attorneys. Dr. Schultz was accused of 'stacking the committee to get the decision the company wanted,' and of falsely stating in an official document that the conclusions reached by the advisory committee were 'clear' and 'unanimous'—to the contrary, they were not. A letter from Senator Grassley to Dr. Torti dated March 6, 2009 indicated that Dr. Schultz and top FDA attorneys had concealed the fact that two of the authors of a major publication presented to the advisory committee in support of the knee implant device, had affiliations with the device manufacturer ('the first author of the article is [the manufacturer's] Vice President of Scientific Affairs,'

Senator Grassley noted).

"Dr. Jay Mabrey, Chief of orthopedic surgery at Baylor University Medical Center in Dallas and Chairman of the advisory committee, should be commended for his integrity and willingness to speak out once he became aware of what had transpired. Dr. Larry Kessler, former Director of the Office of Science and Engineering Laboratories at FDA, who had direct knowledge of the advisory committee meeting and process, characterized the process as 'showing the FDA at its worst.'

"The culture of wrongdoing and cover-up is nothing new but is part of a longstanding pattern of behavior. For example, in July 2005, Dr. Daniel Schultz 'approved a medical device against the unanimous opinion of his scientific staff,' overruling 'more than twenty FDA scientists, medical officers and management staff.' According to the New York Times, the decision represented the first time in the agency's history that a director 'approved a device in the face of unanimous opposition from staff scientists and administrators beneath him.' As described in a Senate Finance Committee report following an investigation led by Senator Grassley, Dr. Schultz never revealed to the public that the FDA scientists, medical officers, and all other staff involved, completely disagreed with his decision. The report also stated that 'what remains the same in FDA's approval of a device or a drug is the requirement that data supporting a sponsor's application for approval be scientifically sound. Otherwise health care providers and insurers as well as patients may question the integrity and reliability of the FDA's assessment of the safety and effectiveness of an approved product' – We completely agree.

"Amazingly, just 3 weeks ago, on March 6, 2009, it was reported by the consumer advocacy organization *Public Citizen* that Dr. Tillman "approved a [medical] device that has failed to demonstrate any clinical benefit" and that showed 'trends toward higher risks of death.' According to *Public Citizen*: 'The March 6, 2009 approval by Dr. Tillman "bears an eerie resemblance to another device, Intergel, an anti-scarring device intended for pelvic surgeries that also demonstrated reduced scarring without clinically validated outcomes. Less than two years after Intergel was approved [by Dr. Schultz], the company removed the product from the market due to reports of post-operative pain, foreign body reactions and tissue scarring requiring repeat surgery, including three deaths among women who received it. This history should have given the FDA pause before once again approving a similar device with a questionable safety record.'

"But now, things may finally change at FDA and meeting the expectations of the public may become a reality. On March 14, 2009, an FDA-wide e-mail was sent from the Acting Secretary of HHS: 'Dr. Margaret 'Peggy' Hamburg will be nominated by the President to serve as the next Commissioner and Dr. Joshua 'Josh' Sharfstein will serve as the Principal Deputy Commissioner of the FDA. The FDA is the premier agency of its kind in the world, and President Obama wants to revitalize the agency and empower it to make the best possible decisions for the American people based on the best science available. Dr. Hamburg and Dr. Sharfstein will work hard to support scientific integrity at FDA, strengthening the ability of the agency's professionals to do their work on behalf of the American people. They are the perfect people to translate the President's vision for the FDA into reality.

"We share your vision and we urge that you provide all necessary support to enable your new leadership to bring change to FDA without delay as part of your planned healthcare reform. As stated in a recent NY Times editorial, you must 'send a clear signal to the bureaucracy that the days of neglect are over.

Officials [must] make clear that the practice of distorting science and weakening regulation to favor industry also is over.' We completely agree.

"FDA must carry out its work in a transparent manner based on sound science in order to improve the lives of all Americans, reduce health care costs, and expand health care access. Much work remains to be done at FDA and all pending matters need to be addressed. The wrongdoing revealed in the Wall Street Journal involves top FDA officials and requires immediate investigation. Astoundingly, since May 2008, Dr. von Eschenbach, Dr. Torti, Mr. McConagha, and numerous top FDA officials, have been well-aware of other serious wrongdoing, and failed to take any actions, while the physicians and scientists who spoke out and refused to comply have suffered retaliation.

"The clearance/approval of medical devices that were not made in accordance with the laws, rules and regulations, need to be re-visited. Furthermore, those FDA employees who have engaged in wrongdoing, who have violated laws, rules, and regulations, who have abused their power and authority, and/or who have engaged in retaliation, should be dealt with swiftly. Immediate and decisive disciplinary action will send a strong message FDA-wide that wrongdoing will no longer be tolerated and those who engage in wrongdoing will be held accountable. Some wrongdoing may be beyond the scope of FDA's jurisdiction and may need referral to the U.S. Attorney General.

All FDA employees who are committed to public integrity, who follow the laws, rules and regulations, who use science to promote public safety and health, and who have the courage and patriotism to speak out, must be protected and must have their professional lives restored. We ask that you accept nothing else."

Now What?

The frightening aspect of these revelations is that every medical device and drug that has been approved over at least the last twenty years has to be recalled because there is no way for anyone to determine which products are on the market today because of widespread fraud and corruption of the FDA decision making process through bribery and extortion. This mind-numbing exposé begs the question, "How has Obama and the Congress addressed the clear and present danger to public safety and national security in the entire well-publicized process of health care reform legislation?" Was the confidence and hope in Obama for serious reforms in bringing the criminals to justice for their heinous acts that the whistleblowers expressed misplaced? How many FDA managers were arrested or even fired since Obama took office?

The answer is that Obama and his minions, having to face the unthinkable prospect that the efficacy and safety of all drug products and medical devices on the market today is suspect, they chose to give the FDA pariahs and Pharmaceutical corporate criminals a free pass. Instead, they attack the insurance industry for their price gouging practices so that the government can take control of dispensing the lethal poisons to trusting unsuspecting senior citizens, born during the American post war baby-boom. Ergo, the very name of the new law, "Patient Protection and Affordable Care Act", while the FDA officials are still running amok, has become the greatest farce in history.

The Congress Inaction

In November of 2007, 14 months before the eruption of

the quiet scandal of the FDA whistleblowers accusing their leadership of criminal conspiracy, bribery, extortion and fraud in issuing most of their approvals for new drugs and medical devices, a congressional subcommittee report found that the FDA had become such a dismal failure that the safety of our food supply, medicines and medical devices was in serious jeopardy. The committee found that the FDA had failed in its mission on all counts[28].

The report begins with the FDA mission statement; "The FDA is responsible for protecting the public health by assuring the safety, efficacy, and security of human and veterinary drugs, biological products, medical devices, our nation's food supply, cosmetics, and products that emit radiation. The FDA is also responsible for advancing the public health by helping to speed innovations that make medicines and foods more effective, safer, and more affordable; and helping the public get the accurate, science-based information they need to use medicines and foods to improve their health."

The committee expounded the list of failures in a scathing 60-page report charging mismanagement and systemic gross incompetence and dereliction of duty as follows:

1. The FDA cannot fulfill its mission because its scientific base has eroded and its scientific organizational structure is weak.
2. The nation's food supply is at risk. Crisis management in FDA's two food safety centers, Center for Food Safety and Applied Nutrition (CFSAN) and Center for Veterinary Medicine (CVM), has drawn attention and resources away from FDA's ability to develop the science base and

---

[28] "FDA Science and Mission at Risk"
http://www.fda.gov/ohrms/dockets/ac/07/briefing/2007

infrastructure needed to efficiently support innovation in the food industry, provide effective routine surveillance, and conduct emergency outbreak investigation activities to protect the food supply.
3. FDA's inability to keep up with scientific advances means that American lives are at risk. While the world of drug discovery and development has undergone revolutionary change — shifting from cellular to molecular and gene-based approaches — FDA's evaluation methods have remained largely unchanged over the last half century. Likewise, evaluation methods have not kept pace with major advances in medical devices and use of products in combination.
4. The FDA cannot fulfill its mission because its scientific workforce does not have sufficient capacity and capability. FDA's failure to retain and motivate its workforce puts FDA's mission at risk. Inadequately trained scientists are generally risk-averse, and tend to give no decision, a slow decision or, even worse, the wrong decision on regulatory approval or disapproval.
5. The FDA cannot fulfill its mission because its information technology (IT) infrastructure is inadequate. The Subcommittee was extremely disturbed at the state of the FDA IT infrastructure. The IT situation at FDA is problematic at best — and at worst it is dangerous. Many of the FDA systems reside on technology that has been in service beyond the usual life cycle. Systems fail frequently, and even email systems are unstable — most recently during an E. coli food contamination investigation. More importantly, reports of product dangers are not rapidly compared and analyzed, inspectors' reports are still hand written and slow to work their way through the compliance

system, and the system for managing imported products cannot communicate with Customs and other government systems (and often miss significant product arrivals because the system cannot even distinguish, for example, between road salt and table salt).

The subcommittee also provided a list of findings with a plan of correction for each"

Finding: FDA science agenda lacks structure and vision, as well as effective coordination and prioritization.

Recommendation: Institute a new scientific organization with adequate oversight and collaboration with scientists in the private sector to remain current with new discoveries and developments.

Finding: The FDA has substantial recruitment and retention challenges.

Recommendation: The FDA should create a distinctive research culture, take concrete steps to hire more high-quality scientific talent, and create better career ladders.

Finding: The FDA has an inadequate and ineffective program for scientist performance.

Recommendation: The FDA should enhance the program to monitor performance metrics and put the appropriate IT infrastructure in place to track the evolution of those metrics.

Finding: The FDA has inadequate funding for professional development.

Recommendation: FDA should develop and support a strong ongoing professional development program to ensure that staff maintains its scientific competence.

Finding: The FDA has not taken sufficient advantage of external and internal collaborations.

Recommendation: The FDA should strengthen its

collaboration across Centers and with other government agencies. It should appoint a Director of External Collaborations to administer a competitive external grants program.

Finding: The Subcommittee believes that there is evidence of important, but slow, progress to improve information sciences and technology at the FDA over the past few years, yet significant gaps remain.

Recommendation: Based on the evidence of important foundational work to date in IT [information technology] and yet the continued existence of critical IT capability gaps, there should be significant investment in IT at the FDA to accelerate progress toward an information processing and communications capability that can support all regulatory science.

Finding: The FDA lacks the information science capability and information infrastructure to fulfill its regulatory mandate.

Recommendation: FDA IT must develop the intramural capability to support all regulatory science activities and should catalyze the development of multi-sectorial shared health information exchanges to support industry innovation and fulfillment of regulatory responsibilities.

Finding: The FDA cannot provide the information infrastructure support to regulate products based on new science.

Recommendation: The FDA must develop the capability to innovate in information science and technology to better support its regulatory mandate and more specifically to support regulatory activities for new science.

Finding: The FDA IT infrastructure is obsolete, unstable, and lacks sufficient controls to ensure continuity of operations or to provide effective disaster recovery services.

Recommendation: The FDA should identify and

implement high-return enhancements of FDA IT infrastructure.

Finding: The IT workforce is insufficient and suboptimally organized.

Recommendation: Strengthen and organize the IT workforce to ensure that it can support the rapid evolution of the FDA information science and technology infrastructure.

Finding: The FDA has experienced decreasing resources in the face of increasing responsibilities.

Recommendation: The FDA resource gap must be corrected to enable the Agency to fulfill its regulatory mandate.

Finding: Recommendations of excellent FDA reviews are seldom followed.

Recommendation: The Office of the Commissioner should develop and report to the Science Board a comprehensive plan for timely and effective implementation of these recommendations.

In brief, the report from the Subcommittee on Science and Technology was marked "confidential" on every paged and hidden in plain sight on the internet. Furthermore there was not one allegation of criminal misconduct or negligence on the part of FDA leaders and no press conference to publicize the finding that our food supply is in danger of wiping out whole communities and that our supply of medicines and medical devices is untrustworthy as to safety and effectiveness. This has to be the greatest whitewash in the history of the world.

Wrap Up

The shocking revelation about the FDA should really be no big surprise. Pundits and journalists have been trying to crack that case for decades. However, the counter plug to those leaks has always been the fear of being ridiculed for being a conspiracy theorist nut-job. Government inefficiency across the board is a well-known fact; but the type of criminal conspiracy and abuse that goes on at the FDA is stunning. These are the people charged with the safety and well-being of every American man, woman and child. This revelation changes the entire paradigm of medical and nursing practice because before, we used to make the distinction between acceptable risk with informed consent and negligence.

However, now that we understand that most drug approvals were granted based on falsified clinical trial results, the tens of millions of people who die each year of adverse drug reaction and interaction are victims of mass murder for profit. Furthermore, everyone that has ever taken a drug advertised has FDA-approved, having wonderful benefits with rare side effects, and got sick, has likely been a victim of producer fraud and government corruption. Consequently, knowing that something is FDA-approved, which used to give us confidence in a product for relatively safe consumption is utterly worthless. We have reached a point of critical mass in which we cannot trust any prescription and must ask, "What harm will this cause." If the physician tells you not to worry, he or she is either a liar or an ignoramus.

14. The Medicinal Mayhem

The United States has the largest pharmaceutical industry in the world. The total industry revenue for 2009 was about 325 billion dollars. This industry has evolved to the point that the media is now calling it the pharmaceutical biotechnology industry. The development of new drugs has evolved from isolating specific ingredients in plants to molecular engineering in creating chemical reactions within the human body that alter biological functions. There are two types of responses to these chemical reactions: the therapeutic effect and the side effect. The first alleviates one or more symptoms or enhances a body function like increasing urine output, raising or lowering blood pressure, and the like. The side effect is an unintended response, which is usually harmful or fatal.

Thus, the goal of research and development is to elicit the therapeutic effect and learn what harmful side effects are likely to occur and estimate what percentage of consumers would be at risk. Side effects, to name a few, can be anything like damage to vital organs, vomiting and diarrhea, constipation, confusion, disorientation, homicidal behavior, suicidal behavior, mood swings, itching, seizures, migraine headaches, twitching, dystonia[29], hair loss, loss of appetite, and sudden death. In the earlier years of drug development new innovations like Alexander Fleming's discovery of Penicillin in 1928 were so dramatic in saving millions of lives over such a short time, that it spawned a powerful industry that can sell its product at any price and

---

[29] Dystonia is a neurological movement disorder, in which sustained severe muscle contractions cause twisting, repetitive movements and grotesque postures.

virtually own its government regulators through political influence or outright bribery.

Subsequently, the people who pioneered the drug industry became highly motivated to repeatedly reproduce the same dramatic effect on society and they have done so countless times despite that many of their products ended up killing thousands of people with little therapeutic benefits. Obviously, the human drive for survival at any cost provides a powerful demand for pharmaceutical solutions that encourages price gouging under the guise of incorporating research and development costs into the price. Certainly, there have been more than a few great discoveries that have provided fast cures for debilitating and painful diseases like antiviral drugs to eradicate shingles. On the other hand, this type of dramatic innovation, resulting in a legal monopoly yielding windfall profits of billions of dollars, gave rise to rampant industry fraud and government corruption.

The Food and Drug Administration got its start in 1906 to protect the public from unscrupulous activity such as the proliferation of cocaine solutions being sold as cure-all elixirs and became known as "snake oil". The new law of the land was simple; before you claim that a medicine will have a certain effect or provide a cure, you have to prove it scientifically. The other part of the FDA mission was to force manufacturers to identify all ingredients in ingestible products and cosmetics on the label for the consumer to have full disclosure of any potentially harmful ingredients.

Over the last century the FDA became known as a stellar organization and had become a universal worldwide model. Anyone who could claim that their product was FDA-approved would inspire confidence in the user that the item underwent rigorous testing and scrutiny. Simultaneously, however, scandal after scandal erupted, charging fraud and bribery, resulting in multiple deaths and disability. The inexplicable phenomenon is that the FDA reputation would always bounce back after a political charade of pretending to shake the management tree to make the bad apples fall out. Every once in a while, some low-echelon lackeys would have to fall on their swords to take the heat off the bosses who gave the orders to approve various drugs despite obviously bogus test results. Perhaps the idea that FDA approval depends mostly on who pays the most money in bribes and political campaign contributions is so horrifying that people are more willing to live in denial and believe that the new president has eradicated the FDA corruption, when in reality it continues unabated.

However, after the latest rude awakenings of 2007, 2008, and 2009, and after tens of millions of unnecessary deaths over the last 50 years, we have to face the problem and deal with it, because the United States food supply being at risk and proliferation of harmful drugs and devices to millions of people that offer little or no benefit threatens to destroy our society. The root cause of the problem is absolute power and greed. The FDA Commissioner and underlings have complete control over 25% of our economy. They decide what products can be legally marketed in the United States and have the power to remove any product immediately from the market with armed enforcers and they don't even need to have probable cause or a warrant to take action.

Such powers, when used with integrity are necessary to protect us from unknowingly ingesting toxic substances. However, the FDA officials have the power to create instant financial success with billions of dollars in profits and help certain companies eliminate the competition and create monopolies. Therefore, with each decision, the stakes are very high and the name-your-price temptation to use the absolute power of selective enforcement is irresistible.

Time after time, we have seen FDA-approved drugs proliferate on the market with claims of miraculous cures with negligible risk of side effects; only to find out that tens of thousands of people suffered permanent damage, or died after distribution of the new drug with little or no benefit to those who escaped harm. Such catastrophes occurred because the manufacturers presented false reports from bogus clinical trials and bribed FDA officials or used political connections to coerce managers into granting approvals. A few of the notable disasters were the **Diethylstilbestrol** scandal of 1971, the generic drug disgrace of 1989, the Fen-Phen and Redux scams of the 1990's, the **Troglitazone travesty** that Parke-Davis perpetrated between 1996 and 2000, the Ketek drug scandal of 2006 revealing patterns of scientific fraud at the FDA, the attempted Crestor flimflam of 2008, and the revelation of radiation poisoning from CT scans in hospitals across the United States

The DES Disaster

Diethylstilbestrol, more popularly known as "DES", was a synthetic form of estrogen that was created in 1938. The FDA approved it in September 1941. Physicians first prescribed it as a 'miracle drug' to prevent miscarriages in women with such a history. It was also used for many ailments afflicting women such as gonorrheal vaginitis, atrophic vaginitis, menopausal symptoms, and postpartum lactation suppression to prevent breast engorgement. This widespread use remained unchecked for thirty years until doctors began reporting an inexplicable increase in breast cancer among women taking DES and a bizarre spike in the number of young women who developed vaginal and cervical cancer in their late teens and early twenties. Most of these young cancer victims were born to mothers who had taken DES during their first trimester of pregnancy. In 1971, the FDA issued an advisory to doctors not to prescribe DES, but never actually banned this product from the market.

The Generic Drug Scandal of 1989

The FDA had officially adopted a policy of using the "honor system" in dealing with pharmaceutical manufacturers. They accepted research reports of clinical trials funded by the manufacturers without investigating the veracity of the data or questioning the likelihood of biased results. The patent protection laws allow a monopoly on new drug formulas for twenty-five years from the filing time, which is usually thirteen to eighteen years prior to marketing. Thus the pharmaceutical manufacturers have from seven to twelve years of price gouging before competition from generic equivalents brings the prices down. Of course, the first producer to hit the market with the generic drug makes a huge windfall because the price is usually less than half of the original and remains relatively high until more competitors join in.

In 1984, the generic drug industry began to expand rapidly as a result of a legislative deal that provided a mandate for the FDA to approve generic drugs more quickly in return for some patented drugs receiving longer protection. Clinical trials were not required; the generic drug makers only needed to pass a laboratory test to show that their product was close enough in formulation to the original to achieve identical efficacy and level of safety. The word "identical" became a relative term.

Therefore, the coveted first position became a hot commodity for the crooked FDA officials accustomed to operating with no inspector general and no oversight from the Department of Health and Human Services. The big generic drug scandal came to light in 1989 when three officials of the Food and Drug Administration pleaded guilty to receiving bribes, and two generic drug companies admitted to providing false data. Additionally, after yet another scandal involving defective generic drugs for epilepsy, Representative John Dingell said that he'd lost confidence in the industry's integrity and the F.D.A.'s ability to ensure safe drugs.

The subsequent media response was astoundingly blasé. One example was a New Times editorial of October 2, 1989 stating, "Frank Young, the F.D.A. Commissioner, has reorganized the agency's generic drug division and appointed an ombudsman. This is a first step but hardly sufficient. Since its honor system has been so grievously breached, the agency needs to impress all drug companies with its intention of making more thorough checks of the data submitted. So much money is at stake that falsification and bribery are constant dangers."[30] This editor should have denounced Frank Young's action as a farce, rather than calling it a "first step." Furthermore, how would the agency officials make an impression of their intent to checking data more thoroughly when they were taking bribes to accept data without verification?

The Fen-Phen and Redux Conspiracy of the 1990's

---

[30] http://www.nytimes.com/1989/10/02/opinion/the-generic-drug-scandal.html

A drug called Pondimin (fenfluramine) had been on the market since 1973 as a non-habit forming appetite suppressant. It wasn't successful because it caused excessive drowsiness, which interfered with people's daily routines. Then In 1983, a University of Rochester pharmacologist named Michael Weintraub introduced a combination of fenfluramine and phentermine, a stimulant which would counter-balance the drowsiness effect. He ran a four-year study, funded in part by the NIH, on 121 subjects averaging 200 pounds, and found that the combination led to the loss of about 32 pounds on average. As a result of that study being published, in 1992, doctors began prescribing the fenfluramine-phentermine cocktail, or "Fen Phen," as an "off-label" combination; meaning that the FDA has no jurisdiction over what doctors prescribe. However, they did have the power to prohibit the manufacturers of the two drugs from promoting the combination as a diet cocktail. Nonetheless, publicity ensued and the Fen-Phen combination became a new craze while the FDA did nothing to study the possible side effects from a drug interaction.

Meanwhile Aminorex, a drug similar to fenfluramine had caused severe lung damage, yet no one at the FDA expressed any concern that fenfluramine could increase the risk of pulmonary hypertension, which was an often fatal lung disease. In 1994, Wyeth official Fred Wilson had expressed concerns about fenfluramine labeling containing only four cases of pulmonary hypertension when a total of 41 had been observed, but no action was taken until 1996.

In 1995, Wyeth introduced Redux (dexfenfluramine), which it hoped would cause fewer adverse effects. However, the FDA's medical officer, Leo Lutwak, insisted upon a black box warning[31] of pulmonary hypertension risks. After Lutwak refused to approve the drug, FDA management had someone else sign it and approved the drug with no black box warning for marketing in 1996 despite the fact that European regulators were requiring a major warning of pulmonary hypertension risks.

In 1996, a 30-year-old woman developed heart problems after only one month of using the Fen-Phen cocktail; when she died in February 1997 her story made the front page of the Boston Globe[32]. Later, In July 1997, after a technician observed heart abnormalities, researchers at the Mayo Clinic released a report on 24 cases of rare heart valve disease in women who took the Fen-Phen combination.[33] The FDA alerted medical doctors that it had received nine additional reports of the same type, and requested all health care professionals to report any such cases to the agency's Med-Watch program, or to their respective pharmaceutical manufacturers. The FDA subsequently received 66 additional reports of heart valve disease, all primarily associated with Fen-Phen. There were also reports of documented heart-valve problems in patients taking only either fenfluramine or dexfenfluramine. The FDA requested that the manufacturers of fenfluramine and dexfenfluramine stress the potential risk to the heart in the drug labeling and in patient package inserts.

As of 1997, the FDA was continuing to receive reports of

---

[31] Warning of the risk of harmful side effects printed on the label in bold font within a black bordered text box.
[32] Hayward, Ed (May 6, 1997). "Diet to Death"; Boston Herald: p. 1
[33] Connolly HM, Crary JL, McGoon MD, Hensrud DD, Edwards BS, Edwards WD, Schaff HV (August 1997). "Valvular heart disease associated with fenfluramine-phentermine". *The New England Journal of Medicine* **337** (9): 581–8.

cardiac valve damage in persons who had taken these drugs. They finally ordered the two drugs, fenfluramine and dexfenfluramine withdrawn from the market after receiving reports that 30% of all women who had taken either the combination of Fen-Phen or either of the two drugs singularly had abnormal echocardiograms, indicating evidence of heart valve damage. The number of people with heart damage was staggering and the number of deaths is unknown.

Troglitazone travesty

Troglitazone was developed as an anti-diabetic and anti-inflammation drug. A Japanese firm developed it and Parke-Davis introduced it In the United States in the late 1990s. Soon thereafter, an undisclosed association of an idiosyncratic reaction leading to drug-induced hepatitis, causing liver damage came to light. One FDA medical officer John Gueriguian, recommended denying its approval due to the potential high liver toxicity, but his superiors overruled his decision and approved it in January 1997. Subsequently, once the prevalence of adverse liver effects became scandalous, Troglitazone was withdrawn from the United Kingdom market in December 1997, and continued to be sold in the USA until 2000 until the number of reports of drug-induced hepatitis was so large that the FDA officials could no longer cover for their corporate criminal clients. The FDA decision to approve Troglitazone in the first place was an act of criminal negligence at best, but to allow it to remain on the market for three additional years knowingly causing liver damage in thousands of people demonstrated a depraved indifference to human life on the part of FDA officials from 1997 to 2000.

Ketek drug scandal of 2006

In 2004 the FDA management approved the sale of Telithromycin, a broad spectrum antibiotic for respiratory infections over the objections of key safety scientists, Dr. Charles Cooper, Dr. David Ross, Dr. Rosemary Johann-Liang and Dr. David Graham. They based their objections on reports from field investigators that they had repeatedly found that the key clinical trial for the drug, involving 24,000 patients, was fraudulent. The corporate criminals were covering up findings of blurred vision and liver and nervous system toxicity.

In July of 2006, the New York Times reported that David Graham, one of four FDA safety officials concerned about safety of the antibiotic in both adults and children, wrote in an E-mail message to another agency official that the drug's 2004 U.S. approval was in error and should be withdrawn. The drug had been prescribed more than 5 million times bringing in revenue of about 100 million dollars. There were reports of liver failure in fourteen adult patients, four of whom died with another twenty-three sustaining serious liver damage. The actual incidents are unknown because adverse effects from medications are not reportable events and actual damage may not become apparent until years after taking the toxic drug for a relatively short period of time.

In June of 2006, the FDA announced that it completed its safety assessment of Ketek and asked the manufacturer to include warnings of liver toxicity and the increased risk of exacerbation of neurological diseases such as myasthenia gravis. This action came six months after the Annals of Internal

Medicine reported cases of serious liver toxicity[34]. Two years earlier, Dr. Graham wrote in an internal FDA memorandum, published in the above referenced New Times Article, ". . . It's as if every principle governing the review and approval of new drugs was abandoned or suspended where Telithromycin is concerned."

Bupropion and Birth Defects

Bupropion is an antidepressant that is being routinely prescribed to women during the first trimester of pregnancy. The FDA has assigned pregnancy category C regarding the use of this drug, declaring that "Animal reproduction studies have shown an adverse effect on the fetus and there are no adequate and well-controlled studies in humans, but potential benefits may warrant use of the drug in pregnant women despite potential risks[35]." They approved the marketing of this drug in 2007 as being safe for ingestion during the first trimester of pregnancy. Yet, the category statement is meaningless. It says that the benefits could outweigh the risks, but we have no idea what those risks are. Nevertheless, as of this writing, the FDA continues to allow GlaxoSmithKline to market this potentially dangerous drug with impunity giving doctors and their patients the impression that the benefits are great and the risks are negligible because there is no evidence to tell us what those risks are. However, the statement itself is false. The fact is that there is evidence showing increased risk of Bupropion causing bizarre birth defects when prescribed

---

[34] Clay KD, Hanson JS, Pope SD, Rissmiller RW, Purdum PP 3rd, Banks PM. "Brief communication: severe hepatotoxicity of Telithromycin: three case reports and literature review" – *Annals of Internal Medicine*, PUBMED index 16481451, March 21, 2006

[35] http://en.wikipedia.org/wiki/Pregnancy_category

during the first trimester of pregnancy. The FDA lied again, after receiving a full report of the actual facts, putting pregnant mothers-to-be in danger yet again to boost the profits of the manufacturer. They have become so arrogant that they even lie about reports that are published and readily available on the internet.

The manufacturer published their report stating, "A retrospective database of infants (n=7005) whose mothers were exposed to bupropion in the first trimester and outside of the first trimester failed to reveal an increased risk for congenital malformation, especially cardiovascular malformation." This statement was blatantly false as it directly contradicted the content of the published research data. Furthermore, who in his or her right mind would think that the questionable benefit of chemically masking feelings of depression is worth the risk of a horribly deformed baby?

Nonetheless, doctors are prescribing Bupropion to Pregnant women who suffer from depression during the first trimester telling their patients that the benefit outweighs a negligible risk of birth defects, determined to conclude that if such defects did occur they would have happened anyway. We need to severely question this approach because GlaxoSmithKline, the FDA and prescribing physicians are leading thousands of trusting vulnerable young pregnant mothers toward a potential catastrophe of causing ghastly birth defects with fraud, deception and abuse.

To begin with, the manufacturer, GlaxoSmithKline, set up an international data registry whereby they received reports of the birthing outcomes of 1,507 women who had taken Bupropion during pregnancy. The actual number they were able to follow was 675 pregnancies to full term. They reported to the

FDA and the world that the incidents of miscarriages and birth defects were no higher in this group than in the general population.

However, it isn't clear where the "general population" data came from. The final report of the study states, "Because of the international scope of the Bupropion Pregnancy Registry, the voluntary nature of recruitment and other methods used, there is no directly comparable group of unexposed pregnant women against whom to evaluate the observed prevalence of birth defects in the Registry[36]."

Moreover, out of 675 full term pregnancies, there were 24 horrible birth defects reported that involved malformation of vital organs and limbs with bizarre anomalies, six of which were incompatible with life. The observed proportion of birth defects in pregnancies with prenatal exposure in the first trimester was 24/675 or 3.6%. The percentage of birth defects in two other studies from prior time periods not related to first trimester Bupropion usage were 2.2% and 2.6% respectively. Therefore, the obvious conclusion is that there is a possible increased risk by 1.5% that can be associated with this drug, although in reality it could be much greater since the sample size was too small to say that any of those birth defects occurred naturally. Thus, since the FDA received this report and still assigned Category "C" to this drug, it is painfully obvious that these government-employed graft-guzzling liars are complicit in double-dealing the public by implying that there is no apparent risk during the first trimester. The truth is that the benefit of masking the symptoms of prenatal depression could never justify the risk that one out of every thirty

---

[36] http://pregnancyregistry.gsk.com/documents/bup_report_final_2008.pdf

women who take this nasty drug during the first trimester of pregnancy could be causing a ghastly birth defect in her unborn child.

Finally, this action by the FDA officials to commit fraud, deceit and abuse to bolster the profits of drug manufacturers is nothing new. We have seen this countless times over the last 50 years with scandal after scandal of FDA officials being caught red handed taking bribes and coercing their scientists into verifying blatantly fraudulent research reports or simply ignoring the actual data. Therefore, it seems unconscionable for any doctor to prescribe Bupropion during the first trimester of pregnancy without informing the patient of a serious risk of horrific birth defects that may be incompatible with life. The obvious depravity of the corrupt FDA bosses and their corporate criminal counterparts is striking.

The Crestor Flimflam

In early November of 2008, Reuter's and all the other major news media outlets had become very excited over Crestor, which is a cholesterol-lowering drug produced by AstraZeneca and is within a classification of drugs called "Statins". The manufacturer began a four-year study called "Jupiter" and ended it after two years claiming astounding results:

Reuter has reported, "The 17,802-patient study was stopped more than two years early by independent safety monitors because the benefit from 20 milligrams of Crestor daily was so pronounced -- 142 heart events with Crestor versus 251 on placebo. For every 25 patients treated, one serious heart event was avoided. Heart attacks were cut by 54 percent, strokes by 48 percent and the need for angioplasty or bypass was cut by 46 percent compared with a placebo. Study subjects taking Crestor were also 20 percent less likely to die from any cause, a secondary goal of the trial"[37].

The idea behind all this flimflam is the prior scientific discovery that C-reactive protein (CRP) levels are a better indicator of risk of heart attack than low-density lipoproteins (LDL), also known as "bad cholesterol". Elevated CRP's are an indicator of arterial inflammation, which purportedly increases the risk of heart attack more than LDL's. The makers of Crestor wanted to see if their product would lower CRP's in people with normal cholesterol levels thereby preventing heart attacks in a previously untreated population.

The conclusion made by participating cardiologists is that they could start prescribing Crestor to everybody to prevent fifty percent of all heart attack deaths and twenty percent of deaths from any cause. Notwithstanding that there might have been some merit to the "startling results", this rush to begin prescribing this drug indiscriminately was reckless and a danger to the well-being of an unsuspecting public for several reasons.

First, there is a risk to taking Crestor because there are reported side effects that range from minor discomfort to catastrophic illness and death. The known side effects of Crestor are headache, nausea, vomiting, diarrhea, muscle pain, liver failure, muscle breakdown (rhabdomyolysis) and kidney failure. In fact, Crestor and the other Statins are so potentially injurious to the liver that periodic liver function studies conducted on all patients during administration of this drug is a standard of care and they have to discontinue use if the liver enzyme levels are 300% above normal or baseline[38].

---

[37] http://www.reuters.com/article/idUSTRE4A81LH20081109
[38] http://www.medicinenet.com/rosuvastatin/article.htm

Second, AstraZeneca, the manufacturer of Crestor, the largest selling cholesterol-reducing drug in the world, orchestrated the study and funded it in order to justify new reasons for prescribing it to people with normal cholesterol levels. Of course, a favorable result would exponentially increase the sales of the drug in question because it means that the entire adult population of the world would believe that Crestor is a miraculous life-extending drug. The potential profit is in the trillions with a retail charge of $3.45 per day per person. Therefore, the research had a built-in bias with a strong stake on the part of the investigators in a desired outcome. Hence, the results are highly suspect.

Third, appropriate scientific methodology requires that non-related independent medical researchers repeat the experiment to verify the results. Although the study involved about 18,000 people, we do not know what confounding variables existed or the statistical significance of the findings to rule out the possibility that the difference in the heart attack rates of the treated versus control groups would have occurred anyway. Moreover, we do not know what the subject selection criteria were so this sample may not have been a microcosm of the entire population. Normally in a study involving disease prevention, the sample size has to be much larger than 18,000 and for much longer than two years.

Additionally, Mark A. Hlatky, M.D. in an editorial published in the New England Journal of Medicine[39] warned that before expanding the use of drugs like Crestor the "evidence should be examined critically". Dr. Hlatky noted the significant

---

[39] Hlatky, M.A. (2008). *New England Journal of Medicine*; 359:2280-2282

relative reductions in risk between the control and treated groups, but also pointed out that absolute differences in risk were more clinically important. The author also stated "To understand who might benefit from high-sensitivity C-reactive protein testing, there should be a detailed analysis of how the estimated (and actual) cardiovascular risk of the screened subjects changed on the basis of their high-sensitivity C-reactive protein levels, particularly in relation to generally accepted risk thresholds and in key subgroups such as women." He also warned that there was no data on the benefit of lowering LDL levels to 55 in healthy individuals and no data on the risk of committing healthy individuals to twenty years of drug therapy.

Consequently, in view of the potentially devastating side effects of the drug called Crestor, there is a risk of liver and kidney damage in reducing the risk of heart attack. There is also insufficient evidence to justify indiscriminate prescribing of Crestor to people with normal cholesterol levels. This is not the same as taking low-dose aspirin. While there may be some justification for prescribing Crestor to people with normal cholesterol to treat high CRP levels, the provider owes a duty to the patient to warn of the possible side effects. Furthermore, the prescribing of Crestor for anything other than lowering high LDL's is an off-label use and more research is needed before doctors can be justified in changing the standards of care.

The Crestor Flimflam Exposed

Nine days after I posted the above information in a blog on November 9, 2008 warning that the Crestor feeding frenzy could be a fraud, the New York Times and other media were echoing those sentiments, calling for "caution in the rush to statins." Finally, the truth about the Jupiter study seeped out confirming that the 17,802 in the study group was a small portion of the 90,000 people who applied with some 82,000 excluded for various reasons that the researchers did not publicize.

Additionally, many physicians had since come forward and cautioned that prescribing Crestor or other statins indiscriminately to healthy individuals was dangerous because the benefits were not that clear and the no one could measure the risk of side effects in a study that lasted only two years. Furthermore, the New England Journal of Medicine editorial cited above stated that 120 people would have to take the drug for two years in order to benefit one person. However, to achieve such a benefit for one person out of 120 would require subjecting the entire group to the risk of renal damage and liver toxicity. Therefore, such a change in the standards of medical care was likely to cause more harm than good.

In conclusion, notwithstanding the desire of the Crestor manufacturers to have every human being on the planet swallow their product every day from the cradle to the grave at a cost of $3.45 per day per person, the more intelligent approach to heart attack prevention is diet and exercise. As Hippocrates once said, "Let medicine be your food and food be your medicine." Medicines like Crestor have their value, but doctors should stick to prescribing statins only when indicated by high levels of low-density lipoproteins (LDL). However, the Jupiter study did raise a possibility that people with elevated C-reactive proteins (CRP) in the blood and normal LDL's can benefit from Crestor because that drug also lowers CRP's, which is another heart attack risk factor.

Nonetheless, my recommendation to physicians who want to rush to prescribe Crestor to everyone is to make certain that their malpractice insurance is paid up. However, I have no doubt that AstraZeneca will be successful in receiving approval from the FDA to market Crestor to healthy young adults as a prophylactic against heart disease based entirely on their one flimsy, prematurely terminated and biased clinical study.

The New Dirty Little Secret; CT Scans are Dangerous to your Health

On July 31, 2010 the New York Times published a report of hundreds of patients across several states who have been suffering the after effects of radiation overdose after a CT scan of the head.[40] Most of these people suffered hair loss that matches the exact width of the scan. Many of the victims have also reported other symptoms of excessive radiation like nausea and vomiting. Apparently, the computer system that controls the amount of radiation emitted in the devices allows the operator wide latitude in setting the intensity of the exposure. Therefore, the consumers are being subjected to a high risk of harmful effects of radiation without their knowledge.

Furthermore, the Food and Drug Administration (FDA) officials have received reports of radiation damage caused by CT scans and have done nothing. State regulators seem to be powerless because the hospitals against whom victims filed complaints have claimed that they did not make any errors, thus indicating that they exposed their patients to dangerous levels of radiation on purpose without the patients' knowledge and consent. In one case a hospital in California had increased the radiation exposure 13 times greater than the manufacturer's safe-

---

[40] http://www.nytimes.com/2010/08/01/health/01radiation.html

level recommendation in order to get clearer pictures.

    This situation is an outrage and is clearly a case of criminal negligence on a massive scale. It is also a violation of patients' rights to arbitrarily cause such dangerous exposure without their knowledge and consent and without proper medical justification such as eradicating malignant tumors. The fact that it is happening on such a wide scale with no government intervention is shocking. What is even more shameful is that the named hospital officials are refusing to take responsibility for their assaults. The Associated Press reported that several hospitals in California stated that they have been using GE Health's dosage level recommendations in the cases where the CT scans caused radiation damage. Finally, the FDA's response to all of this chaos was to issue an alert to all hospitals to check their scanner radiation settings, which is stupid since the hospitals are denying that there were any mistakes and that the technicians used the settings set by the radiology department heads. Certainly, the fact that there are so many incidents of radiation poisoning in so many different hospitals suggests that the problem rests with the design of the device and with a lack of understanding among decision makers as to what is a safe versus risky level of radiation. Presently, radiological experts are dumbfounded and FDA government officials are being ineffectual.

    In summary, we have a new scandal that seems to be receiving very little attention in the press with no palpable response from the public or from government officials. Until July 31, 2010 people believed that CT scans were safe and used less radiation than X-rays. Then we found out that the opposite is true and that thousands of people have been needlessly suffering hair loss, nausea and vomiting and the possibility of developing brain cancer. The hospital managers are telling the investigative reporters that they were either following manufacturer's recommendations, or that they made choices in certain cases to increase the radiation dosage to get clearer images. In this writer's professional opinion, it seems that the culprits for the most part are the management personnel at GE Health, other manufacturers and the officials at the FDA. Regarding the former, there apparently aren't sufficient safeguards in the programming by which the technicians set the level of radiation exposure. Concerning the later, the FDA officials are refusing to establish safe radiation parameters and order a recall of the CT scanning devices to cause GE and the other manufacturers to prevent technicians from being able to go beyond the acceptable dose range. Moreover, we need to have a legal standard of patient safety which prohibits exposing patients to harmful radiation doses, with criminal penalties for non-compliance.

Wrap up

Unfortunately, the few scandals related in this chapter that arose from the efforts of investigative reporters and whistleblowers at the FDA are just the tip of the proverbial iceberg. The frightening aspect of these nefarious events is the consistency of the corruption over at least five decades. We have seen evidence of bribery and extortion with a depraved indifference to human life and greed so intense that the perpetrators are oblivious to the fact that they threaten to decimate our society by endangering our food supply and dispensing toxic poisons being sold as life-saving cures. This is the brink of chaos and the fact that it has perpetuated through every administration since Eisenhower and has escaped the scrutiny of at least fifty sessions of congress makes it reasonable to suspect the existence of a shadow government conspiracy. It seems that the ultimate goal is to weaken the power of the United States in favor of world domination by an elite multinational oligarchy.

Alas, the hopes of the last set of whistle blowers who expressed confidence that Obama was finally going to put an end to FDA corruption by reorganizing are dashed. After more than two years of the Obama administration, and the passing of the Patient Protection and Affordable Health Care Act in March, 2010, which failed to address the scandal-ridden den of criminals known as the "FDA", there is nothing to look forward to because every time we think about taking a prescribed or over-the-counter pill for the first time we have to wonder if it's toxic and every time we go for a CT scan we have to worry about radiation sickness. Anyone who still thinks that any FDA-approved product is safe to use is living in a fool's paradise.

15. PPACA – The Roadmap to Chaos

Obamacare Repeal and the Deficit; Which way is up?

The big argument over whether or not to repeal the Patient Protection and Affordable Care Act (PPACA) is based on fear over whether covering an additional 32 million people will create an insurmountable deficit that will bankrupt America and cause social and economic chaos. The Republicans say that PPACA will cause this chaos and the Democrats say that the repeal of PPACA will cause the chaos. Both sides believe that each is fighting to avoid the pending implosion. Both sides are missing the whole point. The budget busting will come from Medicare which makes the whole argument moot. All people over 65 are covered and the ranks of the elderly are growing exponentially with the baby boomers. Therefore, regarding the future financial fiasco, coverage is a non-issue.

As stated previously, the 50 million or so people without health care coverage are currently using the emergency rooms as their primary care because that is the only place they can go. There are no yearly check-ups and no preventive measures. They have to wait until they are sick in order to gain access. The hospitals by law must take them in whether they can pay or not. The Hill-Burton Act requires that the Feds reimburse the hospitals for their uncollected receivables. Therefore, the government has been paying for everybody's health care anyway and at a much higher cost. ER visits cost an average of $1,600 each including blood tests and x-rays. A clinic visit costs about $200 including blood tests and X-rays. Moving people from ER care to clinic care would save billions, so it is moronic to leave anyone out there with no public option. But this savings will be a drop in the bucket compared to increased Medicare hospital expenditures over the next ten years. There is just no way to predict how much it will be. Both sides are arguing the wrong question. We need to focus on people 65 and older on how to make them healthier and make the care more cost effective. One example is people in nursing homes. The way things work now, if a nursing home resident gets a fever; it's off to the hospital. If the stomach tube pops out, it's off to the hospital. If there is a change in mental status, it's off to the hospital. Our Government wastes hundreds of millions of dollars on ambulance and ER services for nothing, when the old folks could receive everything they need there at the nursing home for pennies on the dollar. That's where we need immediate reform in lowering the cost of caring for the elderly. If we don't, when we become elderly the rest of us will pay with our lives for the bureaucratic folly.

Case in point: The nurse at the nursing home finds that 79 year old Sadie has a temperature of 102 degrees Fahrenheit. She calls the doctor and he tells her to contact the ambulance to take Sadie to the nearest hospital with a diagnosis of "fever of unknown origin." When Sadie arrives at the emergency room, the doctor orders a chest X-ray, electrocardiogram, blood chemistry analysis, urinalysis and a blood culture. All tests are negative except for the urine, which shows signs of bladder infection. The nurse inserts a bladder catheter to get a urine culture. Sadie gets admitted for three days and she is given oral antibiotics. The doctor discharges her on the fourth day and has her transferred back to the nursing home. The total bill to Medicare is about $12,500 dollars. Meanwhile, Medicare has to pay $350 per day for the empty bed at the nursing home. This is a typical scenario and each time the entire problem could be treated at the skilled nursing facility. The Medicare and Medicaid payment policies would have to change allowing additional cost reimbursement for acute health problems at the skilled nursing facility (SNF). The SNF's are allowed to treat illness like pneumonia, bladder infection and other acute problems and they can do it effectively, but they refuse because the government won't reimburse them for the additional cost. The end result is the lunacy of paying for empty beds and the high cost of hospital admission. The total cost of treating "Sadie's" bladder infection would have been about $1,000 over the $350 per day that Medicare is spending for basic nursing home care.

In conclusion, the Medicare and Medicaid reimbursement policies regarding senior citizens in nursing homes are wasting billions of dollars per year. The aforementioned case in point is typical of what is happening every day in thousands of nursing homes across the country. Do we need to repeal PPACA? The answer is unequivocally yes! However, we need to rewrite this law to address the issues of patient protection and wasteful spending by repealing policies instituted by corruption and lunacy. In his 2011 State of the Union speech, Obama said that he would welcome suggestions on how to make the PPACA law better, but he showed more interest in covering people's assets than in saving lives.

The 12 Step Program

Proponents of the new health care law, like Families USA, boast of 12 benefits echoing the Whitehouse propaganda, which took up a portion of the 2011 State-of-the-Union address;
1. Ensure that all Americans have access to quality, affordable health care;

2. Create a new, regulated marketplace where consumers can purchase affordable health care;
3. Extend much needed relief to small businesses;
4. Improve Medicare by helping seniors and people with disabilities afford their prescription drugs;
5. Prohibit denials of coverage based on pre-existing conditions;
6. Limit out-of-pocket costs so that Americans have security and peace of mind;
7. Help young adults by requiring insurers to allow all dependents to remain on their parents plan until age 26;
8. Expand Medicaid to millions of low-income Americans;
9. Provide sliding-scale subsidies to make insurance premiums affordable;
10. Hold insurance companies accountable for how our health care dollars are spent;
11. Clamp down on insurance company abuses;
12. Invest in preventive care.

Therefore we need to examine each of these 12 benefits to see just how beneficial they really will become. Will this law really accomplish any of those lofty goals or are we being set up to fall victim in a diabolical scheme to take control of who shall live and who shall die?

... With Liberty and Coverage for all

The claim that PPACA "ensures that all Americans have access to quality, affordable health care," is laughable. The estimates in the latter part of 2010 were that at least 23 million people will not have access to coverage under the new law. Moreover, the issue of patient safety has not been addressed at all, and while health care providers are killing enough people to become the fifth leading cause of death in America, one can hardly call this quality care. Additionally, as to healthcare becoming affordable, the new law encourages large deductibles of $6,000 to $10,000 per person per year for people with pre-existing conditions and $2,000 to $4,000 for healthy folks, thereby blowing affordability to smithereens.

Thus, the commercial health plan has become nothing more than an insurance policy to protect one's assets from the cost of hospitalization. You're betting that you will need hospital care and the insurance company is betting that you won't. In the private insurance market the healthy pay for the sick. If there aren't enough healthy people in the pool, the insurer goes belly up. That's why the new scheme won't work without mandatory coverage.

How much is Affordable?

The insurance exchange scheme for the purchase of "affordable" health care is a shell game. The term "affordable" that keeps popping up is empty and meaningless because there are no price controls in the new law. The Congress makes the false assumption that free market competition will keep prices down. Section 1003 of the new law states:

"The process established under paragraph (1) shall require health insurance issuers to submit to the Secretary and the relevant State a justification for an unreasonable premium increase prior to the implementation of the increase. Such issuers shall prominently post such information on their Internet websites. The Secretary shall ensure the public disclosure of information on such increases and justifications for all health insurance issuers."

This section requires that the insurance providers disclose their intent to gouge the consumers with unreasonable increases in premiums and submit a justification. This clearly indicates that unreasonable premium increases will be tolerated. Take notice that the new law does not define what an "unreasonable increase" is, nor does it tell us under what conditions such increases will be accepted. The Secretary of Health and Human Services has complete discretion and may delegate these powers to anyone of her choosing. If the history of the FDA is any lesson, the door to corruption is wide open and the price gouging will continue unabated.

Small Businesses Owners: Relieved or Reviled?

Regarding the extending of much needed relief to small businesses; I don't know any small business owners who feel relieved. Companies that have less than fifty employees are still not required to provide health benefits and most of them don't. Companies that have fifty or more employees will now have to purchase some form of health plan for their workers, so this drives up the cost of doing business even with the new tax credits. There are three choices, pass the extra cost on to the customers, keep the number of jobs less than fifty or go out of business; in short, higher inflation and fewer jobs.

Drug Coverage for Seniors

The PPACA is supposed to close the so-called doughnut hole by providing more prescription drug coverage. However, the language of this provision is so convoluted that no one can figure out who gets what when. The initial step in this spaghetti bowl is that Section 3315, which called for the immediate reduction in coverage gap in 2010, was repealed and replaced. Thus, the law makers wrote one section and then repealed and replaced it with another without first writing out what they were repealing. Then, the authors added Section 1101 of Subtitle "B" – Medicare to first close the drug coverage gap in 2010 as follows:

"(c) Coverage gap rebate for 2010.— (1) in general—In the case of an individual described in subparagraphs (A) through (D) of section 1860D–14A(g)(1) who as of the last day of a calendar quarter in 2010 has incurred costs for covered part D drugs so that the individual has exceeded the initial coverage limit under section 1860D–2(b)(3) for 2010, the Secretary shall provide for payment from the Medicare Prescription Drug Account of $250 to the individual by not later than the 15th day of the third month following the end of such quarter."

In case anyone could figure out if they qualify as being the types of people described in subparagraphs (A) through (D) of section 1860D–14A(g)(1), they were supposed to receive a $250 rebate if they spent more than that for out-pocket costs on covered drugs. In any event, 2010 has come and gone as of this writing in 2012, so this subsection 1101 has timed out and is no longer relevant. Moreover, for most seniors, the process of filing for and collecting such a rebate without being able to figure out who is eligible is insurmountable. Uncle Sam might as well have put the $250 on top of Mount Everest and told the elderly folks to go fetch it.

Starting in 2011, eligible individuals are supposed to receive a discount of 7% of out-of-pocket costs on applicable medications which will increase by 7% each year until it reaches 75% by 2020. Again, the seniors will have to jump through fire hoops just to find out if they are eligible.

Covering Pre-existing Conditions with Conditions: "Let them Eat Deductibles"

From its inception until 2014, the PPACA law establishes a high risk pool for people with pre-existing conditions. If you have a long-standing chronic disease like diabetes, well controlled, with no complications, you will be counted as a high risk for future high cost expenditures. The penalty for having treatable medical conditions when buying coverage is, having to eat a whopping six to ten thousand dollar deductible. Thus the entire cost for keeping a chronic condition like high blood pressure under control is on the health care consumer. The six hundred dollar per month premium is to pay for hospital care and rehabilitation in case of a catastrophic event, like a stroke or heart attack. Therefore, the highly publicized elimination of the pre-existing condition exclusions is a charade. Moreover, the out-of-pocket burden discourages the person from seeking preventive care because the affordable care is too expensive to manage pre-existing conditions.

For the rest of time after the 2014 change-over, PPACA makes some vague confusing reference to pre-existing conditions in the "Level Playing Field" section as follows: "(a) IN GENERAL.—*as revised by section 10104(n)*. Notwithstanding any other provision of law, any health insurance coverage offered by a private health insurance issuer shall not be subject to any Federal or State law described in subsection (b) if a qualified health plan offered under the Consumer Operated and Oriented Plan program under section 1322, or a multi-State qualified health plan under section 1334, is not subject to such law." What this means is anybody's guess. I would like to know what the authors of this statute were smoking at the time.

The actual plan is to force everybody to purchase health care coverage so that the young and healthy can pay for the care provided to those with pre-existing conditions. The statute itself under section 1501, "Individual Responsibility" states that Congress finds that the success of this entire venture depends entirely upon mandatory health coverage purchase. "(I) under sections 2704 and 2705 of the Public Health Service Act (as added by section 1201 of this Act), if there were no requirement, many individuals would wait to purchase health insurance until they needed care. By significantly increasing health insurance coverage, the requirement, together with the other provisions of this Act, will minimize this adverse selection and broaden the health insurance risk pool to include healthy individuals, which will lower health insurance premiums. The requirement is essential to creating effective health insurance markets in which improved health insurance products that are guaranteed issue and do not exclude coverage of preexisting conditions can be sold."

Therefore, the success of the entire legislative action is dependent upon all healthy citizens and residents of the U.S. purchasing a health plan on the insurance exchange. Since the U.S. Supreme Court ruled that the $750 non-purchase penalty is a tax and therefore constitutional, all of the healthy people now have the choice of paying $4,000 annually in premiums with a $6,000 deductible or $750 as an add-on tax with no coverage. Why would they choose the insurance and still have to pay the first $6,000 in costs? It would be much cheaper to pay the $750 tax and wait until they have an emergency. Then they can still purchase a health plan on the way to the hospital from their smart phones on the insurance exchange or while waiting in the emergency room for a diagnosis. As long as the purchase takes place before the rendering of a diagnosis there is no pre-existing condition. And even if the purchase takes place after diagnosis and admission, the purchaser simply moves into the high-risk pool and pays a higher premium; it's still a lot cheaper than paying the hospital bills directly. You don't have to be a genius to figure out which is the better deal.

The Outer Limits of Out-of-Pocket Costs

Obama said we can all breathe a sigh of relief because PPACA is going to limit our out-of-pocket health care costs with monstrous deductibles. Starting with the high risk pools, this is what the new law says about limiting out of pocket expenses:

"(A) provides to all eligible individuals health insurance coverage that does not impose any preexisting condition exclusion with respect to such coverage; (B) provides health insurance coverage—(i) in which the issuer's share of the total allowed costs of benefits provided under such coverage is not less than 65 percent of such costs; and (ii) that has an out of pocket limit not greater than the applicable amount described in section 223(c)(2) of the Internal Revenue Code of 1986 for the year involved, except that the Secretary may modify such limit if necessary to ensure the pool meets the actuarial value limit under clause (i); (C) ensures that with respect to the premium rate charged for health insurance coverage offered to eligible individuals through the high risk pool, such rate shall—(i) except as provided in clause (ii), vary only as provided for under section 2701 of the Public Health Service Act (as amended by this Act and notwithstanding the date on which such amendments take effect); (ii) vary on the basis of age by a factor of not greater than 4 to 1; and (iii) be established at a standard rate for a standard population; and (D) meets any other requirements determined appropriate by the Secretary."

In other words, for people under the age of sixty-five with pre-existing conditions, the out-pocket-costs will be limited only to the extent that the health insurance companies can still remain profitable as the Secretary of Health and Human Services shall determine. Furthermore, there are no anti-gouging provisions regarding what the physicians and hospitals can charge consumers for non-covered services. To wit, a private hospital can still gouge us for $10,000 for a three-day hospital stay to cover the deductible even though Medicare would have paid only $3,500. Hence, those of us under sixty-five years of age who have a pre-existing condition are left with assured coverage that costs more than housing in this new affordable health care system. Therefore, while having no coverage leaves us at risk of falling into poverty from medical bills, under the new law, poverty is guaranteed, unless the person in this scenario is smart enough to delay purchasing coverage until he/she needs to go to the hospital.

Regarding the rest of the under sixty-five years of age out-of-pocket population, there is some confusing language about forcing the insurance companies to reduce out-of-pocket cost sharing such as co-pays for families whose income is 100%, 200% and 300% of poverty level by two thirds, one half and one third respectively.

"SEC.1402. REDUCED COST-SHARING FOR INDIVIDUALS ENROLLING (a) IN GENERAL.—In the case of an eligible insured enrolled in a qualified health plan—(1) the Secretary shall notify the issuer of the plan of such eligibility; and (2) the issuer shall reduce the cost-sharing under the plan at the level and in the manner specified in subsection (c). (b) ELIGIBLE INSURED.—In this section, the term "eligible insured" means an individual— (1) who enrolls in a qualified health plan in the silver level of coverage in the individual market offered through an Exchange; and (2) whose household income exceeds 100 percent but does not exceed 400 percent of the poverty line for a family of the size involved. In the case of an individual described in section 36B(c)(1)(B) of the Internal Revenue Code of 1986, the individual shall be treated as having household income equal to 100 percent for purposes of applying this section. (c) DETERMINATION OF REDUCTION IN COST-SHARING.—(1) REDUCTION IN OUT-OF-POCKET LIMIT.—(A) IN GENERAL.—The reduction in cost-sharing under this subsection shall first be achieved by reducing the applicable out-of pocket limit under section 1302(c)(1) in the case of—(i) an eligible insured whose household income is more than 100 percent but not more than 200 percent of the poverty line for a family of the size involved, by two-thirds; (ii) an eligible insured whose household income is more than 200 percent but not more than 300 percent of the poverty line for a family of the size involved, by one-half; and (iii) an eligible insured whose household income is more than 300 percent but not more than 400 percent of the poverty line for a family of the size involved, by one-third."

The Independent Dependents

When hearing about extending the cutoff age for covered dependent children, it seems simple and straight forward until we read that the law provides for the Secretary of Health and Human Services to have discretion over defining whether a child is "dependent" or not.

"SEC. 2714. EXTENSION OF DEPENDENT COVERAGE (a) IN GENERAL.—A group health plan and a health insurance issuer offering group or individual health insurance coverage that provides dependent coverage of children shall continue to make such coverage available for an adult child until the child turns 26 years of age. Nothing in this section shall require a health plan or a health insurance issuer described in the preceding sentence to make coverage available for a child of a child receiving dependent coverage as *revised by section 2301(b) of HCERA*. (b) REGULATIONS.—The Secretary shall promulgate regulations to define the dependents to which coverage shall be made available under subsection (a). (c) RULE OF CONSTRUCTION.—Nothing in this section shall be construed to modify the definition of 'dependent' as used in the Internal Revenue Code of 1986 with respect to the tax treatment of the cost of coverage."

Furthermore, since grandchildren are not included in family covered at any age, this law causes a gap in coverage for children who are living with their grandparents and don't qualify under the Child Health Insurance Program law (CHIP).

The Medicaid Stretch

The "poverty line", which determines access to health care, is an arbitrary per capita income level. If a person's income is even one penny above this number he or she is not eligible for Medicaid. This is why we have full time workers in the United States who have no access to health care until they suffer from acute illness and need emergency treatment. The consequences are obvious and devastating; millions of people dying of treatable illness every year.

To wit, the problem is the cutoff. Medicaid is totally free for those people under sixty-five years of age who are destitute with zero net worth and there is no provision for a non-eligible individual to pay for coverage because that would cause an intolerable state of competition between private industry and government. That was the argument that convinced Congress to eliminate the so called "public option" that would have finally closed this gap.

Moreover, the Medicaid expansion provision in this law (Title II, Subtitle A; "Improved Access to Medicaid) has moved the cutoff line to include about ten million more people whose income is up to 133 percent above the current poverty line. However, there is still no coverage for most of the uncovered in the financially deprived segment of American society. Therefore, the health care reform law has failed to meet its stated goal of providing access to health care for all Americans. The problem is that there is a new cutoff which literally still cuts off 23 million Americans from having access to health care outside of the emergency room.

Sliding Scale on a Slippery Slope

The sliding scale idea of reducing the cost of health insurance through tax credits is useless because the consumer must first purchase the insurance and pay the bloated premium and wait until the end of the year for the tax break. That does nothing to relieve the burden of having to sacrifice other necessities to pay for insurance just in case something might happen in the future. Moreover, to add another hurdle to an already impossible situation, Congress decided to make it impossible to figure out the amount of the tax credit subsidy with more confusing language that sounds like a brain teaser riddle. Note the following:

"(1) IN GENERAL.—The term 'premium assistance credit amount' means, with respect to any taxable year, the sum of the premium assistance amounts determined under paragraph (2) with respect to all coverage months of the taxpayer occurring during the taxable year.

"(2) PREMIUM ASSISTANCE AMOUNT.—The premium assistance amount determined under this subsection with respect to any coverage month is the amount equal to the lesser of—(A) the monthly premiums for such month for 1 or more qualified health plans offered in the individual market within a State which cover the taxpayer, the taxpayer's spouse, or any dependent (as defined in section 152) of the taxpayer and which were enrolled in through an Exchange established by the State under 1311 of the Patient Protection and Affordable Care Act, or (B) the excess (if any) of—(i) the adjusted monthly premium for such month for the applicable second lowest cost silver plan with respect to the taxpayer, over (ii) an amount equal to 1/12 of the product of the applicable percentage and the taxpayer's household income for the taxable year.

"(3) OTHER TERMS AND RULES RELATING TO PREMIUM ASSISTANCE AMOUNTS.—For purposes of paragraph (2)—(A) APPLICABLE PERCENTAGE.—(i) IN GENERAL.—a*s revised by section 1001(a)(1)(A) of HCERA.* Except as provided in clause (ii), the applicable percentage for any taxable year shall be the percentage such that the applicable percentage for any taxpayer whose household income is within an income tier specified in the following table shall increase, on a sliding scale in a linear manner, from the initial premium percentage to the final premium percentage specified in such table for such income tier:

"In the case of household income (expressed as a percent of poverty line) within the following income tier:	The initial premium percentage is—	The final premium percentage is—
Up to 133%	2.0%	2.0%
133% up to 150%	3.0%	4.0%
150% up to 200%	4.0%	6.3%
200% up to 250%	6.3%	8.05%
250% up to 300%	8.05%	9.5%
300% up to 400%	9.5%	9.5%

"(ii) INDEXING.—as *added by section 1001(a)(1)(B) of HCERA instead of clauses (ii) and (iii) previously here.*

"(I) IN GENERAL.—Subject to sub clause (II), in the

case of taxable years beginning in any calendar year after 2014, the initial and final applicable percentages under clause (i) (as in effect for the preceding calendar year after application of this clause) shall be adjusted to reflect the excess of the rate of premium growth for the preceding calendar year over the rate of income growth for the preceding calendar year.

"(II) ADDITIONAL ADJUSTMENT.—Except as provided in sub clause (III), in the case of any calendar year after 2018, the percentages described in sub clause (I) shall, in addition to the adjustment under sub clause (I), be adjusted to reflect the excess (if any) of the rate of premium growth estimated under sub clause (I) for the preceding calendar year over the rate of growth in the consumer price index for the preceding calendar year.

"(III) FAILSAFE.—Sub clause (II) shall apply for any calendar year only if the aggregate amount of premium tax credits under this section and cost-sharing reductions under section 1402 of the Patient Protection and Affordable Care Act for the preceding calendar year exceeds an amount equal to 0.504 percent of the gross domestic product for the preceding calendar year."

Thus the tax credit idea does nothing to provide access to health care to those defined as "the working poor."

The main problem with attempting to make health care affordable is that there is no definition of "affordable health care." It really comes down to answering the question of what percentage of income should we consider reasonable to spend on all of our health care needs. If you take a survey, I'm certain you will get a wide range of answers. On the whole, we spend 26 percent of our GDP on health care products and services. That's 26 cents of every dollar that we spend on everything that we buy.

We all have a sense of priority based on what we need now to survive. We will spend whatever we have to stay alive and relieve pain and suffering when we face catastrophic illness or injury.

However, as we go through our daily activities in reasonably good health we will focus on obtaining food, maintaining shelter with comfortable climactic conditions, transportation and staying connected with telephones and internet access. Health care is only a potential necessity that receives low priority until we actually need it. Consequently, while the potential for financial ruin due to catastrophic illness looms large for all thinking individuals, if the cost of protection itself causes financial deprivation, the motivation for buying such an insurance product wanes. Hence, the question, "What percentage of income is reasonable to spend on health insurance?" The answer depends on the amount of total income. If one is spending 100 percent on food, shelter, transportation and communication with no disposable income, what does he or she have to give up while paying premiums with high deductibles? Should we skip meals or allow our car insurance to lapse? Maybe we can tell the landlord or mortgage holder, "Sorry I have to skip this month's payment because I have to pay for my health insurance and I still need money for the doctor's visits."

Therefore, we need to come to a consensus of what is a reasonable percentage of income to allocate to health insurance. Should we be required to make life-style adjustments and move to poorer neighborhoods with substandard housing to be able to purchase a health plan? I don't think anyone will sanction that, especially when the insured population still has to pay out of pocket for routine medical services because of the co-pays and humongous deductibles. As stated previously, the regular person pays an average of $1,500 per year on health care over a lifetime.

If we have to pay more than that in premiums and still get stuck with co-pays and deductibles it's a rip-off.

Finally, we come to the issue of price gouging uninsured individuals. Why do hospitals have the right to charge uncovered individuals 300 percent over what they accept from health plans for the same services? Why does a doctor have the right to charge me $150 for a fifteen minute visit when he or she accepts $59 from an insurance company or a preferred provider organization (PPO) for the same service?

Holding Insurance Companies accountable for how our health care dollars are spent

It's difficult to ascertain what authority the U.S. government has to dictate to a private company how to spend its revenue. One would think that there is no such power at any level. However government does have the power to levy special taxes against any industry that is reaping a windfall. In that sense congress can provide incentives for insurance companies to reduce their administrative overhead and spend more on actual health care by making the pre-approval process less cumbersome for the consumer. But that would never happen in Congress because it makes sense. Instead, the Congressional law writers decided to hatch another hair-brained scheme hoping to manipulate the free market to do its bidding. Paragraph "J" in Section 1501 says, "Administrative costs for private health insurance, which were $90,000,000,000 in 2006, are 26 to 30 percent of premiums in the current individual and small group markets. By significantly increasing health insurance coverage and the size of purchasing pools, which will increase economies of scale, the requirement, together with the other provisions of this Act, will significantly reduce administrative costs and lower health insurance premiums. The requirement is essential to creating effective health insurance markets that do not require underwriting and eliminate its associated administrative costs."

Thus, the Congressional law writers believe that forcing everyone to purchase health insurance starting January 2, 2013 will bring about a larger pool on which to spread the risk and will somehow magically reduce the administrative cost allocations. Of course, the top corporate executives will slash their salaries just to make sure that Obamacare works.

Clamping Down on Insurance Abuses?

The way that insurance companies have been able to abuse their customers is by requiring prior authorization for specialty referrals, diagnostic tests, elective surgery, emergency room visits, brand name medication for which there is no cheaper generic substitute, surgical supplies and durable medical equipment. Most of these prior approval requests are judged on the basis of medical necessity determined by the results of a computer program analysis which requires a staff of registered nurses and physicians to give the automated denial the appearance of credibility. Thus, the insurance company has the absolute right to deny coverage for any prescribed diagnostic procedure or treatment declaring that it is not medically necessary. The right to appeal means nothing because the time it takes to complete that process renders the issue moot.

Notwithstanding that precertification allows insurance companies to control cost by preventing treatment and does nothing to lower cost to consumers, the PPACA eliminates prior approval only for pediatrics, obstetrics and gynecology and emergency room visits in Section 2719A—Patient Protections. The preauthorization process remains in effect for all other forms of health care. Hence, the new law clamps down more on consumers than it does on health insurance providers.

Prevention Intervention Investments

Finally, to fulfill the promise of more investment in preventive care, SEC. 399U of PPACA establishes the Community Preventive Services Task Force (CPSTF). Of course, this is not to be confused with the pre-existing U.S. Preventive Services Task Force (USPSTF) and the Advisory Committee on Immunization Practices (ACIP). Aside from the obvious duplications, the duties and responsibilities of the CPSTF are absurd.

"(a) ESTABLISHMENT AND PURPOSE.—The Director of the Centers for Disease Control and Prevention shall convene an independent Community Preventive Services Task Force (referred to in this subsection as the 'Task Force') to be composed of individuals with appropriate expertise. Such Task Force shall review the scientific evidence related to the effectiveness, appropriateness, and cost-effectiveness of community preventive interventions for the purpose of developing recommendations, to be published in the Guide to Community Preventive Services (referred to in this section as the 'Guide'), for individuals and organizations delivering population-based services, including primary care professionals, health care systems, professional societies, employers, community organizations, non-profit organizations, schools, governmental public health agencies, Indian tribes, tribal organizations and urban Indian organizations, medical groups, Congress and other policymakers. Community preventive services include any policies, programs, processes or activities designed to affect or otherwise affecting health at the population level.

"(b) DUTIES.—The duties of the Task Force shall include—(1) the development of additional topic areas for new recommendations and interventions related to those topic areas, including those related to specific populations and age groups, as well as the social, economic and physical environments that can have broad effects on the health and disease of populations and health disparities among sub-populations and age groups; (2) at least once during every 5-year period, review interventions and update recommendations related to existing topic areas, including new or improved techniques to assess the health effects of interventions, including health impact assessment and population health modeling; (3) improved integration with Federal Government health objectives and related target setting for health improvement; (4) the enhanced dissemination of recommendations; (5) the provision of technical assistance to those health care professionals, agencies, and organizations that request help in implementing the Guide recommendations; and (6) providing yearly reports to Congress and related agencies identifying gaps in research and recommending priority areas that deserve further examination, including areas related to populations and age groups not adequately addressed by current recommendations.

(c) ROLE OF AGENCY—The Director shall provide ongoing administrative, research, and technical support for the operations of the Task Force, including coordinating and supporting the dissemination of the recommendations of the Task Force, ensuring adequate staff resources, and assistance to those organizations requesting it for implementation of Guide recommendations.

"(d) COORDINATION WITH PREVENTIVE SERVICES TASK FORCE—The Task Force shall take appropriate steps to coordinate its work with the U.S. Preventive Services Task Force and the Advisory Committee on Immunization Practices, including the examination of how each task force's recommendations interact at the nexus of clinic and community.

"(e) OPERATION—in carrying out the duties under subsection (b), the Task Force shall not be subject to the provisions of Appendix 2 of title 5, United States Code.

"(f) AUTHORIZATION OF APPROPRIATIONS—there are authorized to be appropriated such sums as may be necessary for each fiscal year to carry out the activities of the Task Force."

Although on the surface it appears that there is a provision for investing in preventive health research, it really does nothing more than create yet another superfluous bureaucracy to funnel large sums of cash to political contributors for more redundant studies and useless recommendations.

Wrap up

In summary, we have seen that the PPACA is a dismal failure. Wasteful spending will continue unabated, especially in the unnecessary hospitalization of patients in skilled nursing facilities because the new law simply does not address it. The idea of patient protection is a joke because there is no provision for establishing patient safety standards. As for access to affordable quality care for all Americans, anyone who still believes in Obamacare is a bit late for his/her next dose of medication.

Twenty-three million Americans will still have no access to coverage, so many of them will have to die of treatable diseases and the hospitals will continue to kill twenty-two people every hour by accident; so what good is the new law if it's going to bankrupt America and not save any more lives?

Additionally, the PPACA statute is mostly indecipherable, like the ramblings of a lunatic. It is so convoluted that we have to consult several other laws to figure out how to qualify for benefits that don't exist. For those benefits that do exist if there are any, we find that only Tibetan Monks who have successfully meditated on the peak of Mt. Everest for at least three years with no food or water can qualify.

16. New National Priorities for Health Care Reform

With all of the chaos amid the bogus health reform movement, the irony of the last two decades is that within the bureaucratic morass of committees and reports there are cogent solutions to stem the tide of spiraling health care costs, eliminate disparities and improve the quality of care. There were recently published recommendations for the political leadership to take certain actions that would actually work out the health care issues and prevent the impending economic blowout without resorting to inhumane rationing death panels. Thus far, the previous and current administrations have either been shielded from common sense or chose to ignore it. In any event, these proposals are still there as part of the public record and in this chapter we shall explore those to see how easily our Government leaders can reset our national priorities to actually resolve the health care crisis.

The Future Directions Committee can Save the Day

In April of 2010, Harvey V. Fineberg, M.D., Ph.D., president of the Institute of Medicine (IOM) had this to say: "Ten years after the publication of the Institute of Medicine's landmark Quality Chasm series of reports, we often do not know to what extent quality of care has improved. A range of studies and reports indicate that the quality of health care received in our nation is less than optimal, but we continue to lack sufficient information to determine how well new programs, changes in processes, and other interventions improve the quality and equity of care[41]."

Thereby, Dr. Fineberg headed an elaborate and expensive effort to constructing a report on how to write reports about improving quality. It seems that now a web of committees exists to evaluate the types of data needed to evaluate trends in health care screw-ups and disparities. Moreover, Dr. Fineberg made a statement of the colossal failure of the Government's "effort" to improve patient safety and reduce disparities as follows:

"As the United States continues to devote extensive resources toward achieving a high-value, high-quality health care system, the capacity to evaluate the state of care is increasingly important. Since 2003, the annual publication of the National Healthcare Quality Report (NHQR) and National Healthcare Disparities Report (NHDR) by the Agency for Healthcare Research and Quality (AHRQ) has played an important role in documenting trend data on the state of health care quality and disparities. The general message from the most recent reports is that while some areas have improved, the overall quality of health care in the United States is suboptimal. Across all of the process of care measures tracked in the NHQR, persons received the recommended care less than 60 percent of the time. Furthermore, even when quality has improved on a measure tracked in the NHQR, disparities in care often persist across socioeconomic groups, racial and ethnic groups, and geographic areas[42]."

However, the surprising element here is that in April of 2010, one month after Congress passed PPACA, Dr. Fineberg and his Institute of Medicine staff issued a report entitled "Future

---

[41] http://www.ahrq.gov/research/iomqrdrreport/futureqrdrpre.htm#Reviewers
[42] http://www.ahrq.gov/research/iomqrdrreport/futureqrdrsum.htm#ahrq9a

Directions for the National Healthcare Quality and Disparities Reports" with the stated purpose of improving the quality and effectiveness of the information contained in the AHRQ's two major publications; the NHQR and NHDR. During the aforementioned initiative, the IOM formed the ad hoc Future Directions Committee (FDC) which, as a byproduct, also recommended new national priorities in health care reform as follows:

1. **Patient and family engagement:** Engage patients and their families in managing their health and making decisions about their care.
2. **Population health:** Improve the health of the population.
3. **Safety:** Improve the safety and reliability of the U.S. health care system.
4. **Care coordination:** Ensure patients receive well-coordinated care within and across all health care organizations, settings, and levels of care.
5. **Palliative care:** Guarantee appropriate and compassionate care for patients with life-limiting illnesses.
6. **Overuse:** Eliminate overuse while ensuring the delivery of appropriate care.
7. **Access:** Ensure that care is accessible and affordable for all segments of the U.S. population.
8. **Health systems infrastructure capabilities:** Improve the foundation of health care systems (including infrastructure for data and quality improvement; communication across settings for coordination of care; and workforce capacity and distribution among other elements) to support high-quality care.

These national priority recommendations, although

bearing some resemblance to the political rhetoric of the last two years, seem lost in obscurity amid the frenzy over a health system that is choking the life out of our economy and has itself become the fifth leading cause of death in America. Thus, given that the above list is how real health care reform should look, the next logical step is to work out the details on how to accomplish these goals and present them to the appropriate Congressional committees. Rather than a futile attempt at total repeal, what would make more sense is to drastically alter PPACA to simplify the language, eliminate the ambiguities, resolve the constitutional issues and incorporate what's missing to establish patient safety standards and include all Americans in the coverage umbrella. In short, the law needs a major rewrite, but it is doable.

However, the above incisive propositions thus far have gone unheeded because our political leaders would have to make decisions that would set aside special interests in favor of what is best for the American people as a whole. Therefore, in the face of a lackluster Republican Party opposition and a gridlocked Congress, the implementation will have to be left to a grassroots political activist movement such as the "Tea Party." Nonetheless, we shall now explore each of the above proposed national goals and how to achieve them.

Patient and Family Engagement—Informed Consent

First, there must be a mandate for health care providers to include patients and their family members or significant others as partners in the decision making process. There is no one more attached to achieving the best possible outcome than the patient and his or her loved ones. Therefore, when we have information that we can process, we will all choose a course of treatment we believe to be the best chance for recovery with the least risk of harm. Therefore, patient education with the aim of obtaining informed consent is the key.

However, some choices are indeed difficult. Medical judgment is mostly "Let's try this and hope for the best." Doctors prescribe treatments on the basis of FDA approval, manufacturer marketing and what other doctors are prescribing for similar conditions. All the while, they knowingly or unknowingly rely on a corrupt system replete with collusion, bribery and coercion of employees who try to operate with integrity. Scientific evidence is supposed to play a significant role, but unfortunately, almost all clinical trials of drugs and devices are funded by manufacturers who have a vested interest in a favorable result.

Moreover, the IOM published a report in 2004 entitled "Health Literacy: A Prescription to End Confusion" in which it identified health illiteracy as a root cause of treatment failure and complications causing survivable injury and death. The report states that "nearly half of all American adults—90 million people—have difficulty understanding and acting upon health information[43]." So, 90 million adults and their children are at the mercy of the fragmented, confusing and corrupted health care system. What's more, they don't even understand how to provide an accurate health history on which doctors base fifty percent of their diagnoses.

Therefore, the revised health care reform law must

---

[43] Health Literacy: A Prescription to End Confusion; Committee on Health Literacy (Author), Lynn Nielsen-Bohlman (Editor), Allison M. Panzer (Editor), David A. Kindig (Editor); National Academies Press; 1st edition (June 30, 2004)

include a mandate requiring that all medical care providers obtain informed consent before prescribing any treatment. This puts the onus on the physician to provide complete information that lay people can understand. The elements that define "informed consent" must include the following information in lay terms with patient or significant other with acknowledgment of understanding:

1. The patient's diagnosis, with an explanation in lay terms of how the disease affects body functions;
2. The nature and purpose of a proposed treatment or procedure and how it is to be administered;
3. The possible side effects or complications of a proposed treatment or procedure;
4. The risks of not receiving or undergoing a treatment or procedure;
5. Options for alternative treatments or procedures (regardless of their cost or the extent to which other options are covered by health insurance);
6. The nature and benefits of the alternative treatments or procedures;
7. The risks of side effects or complications from alternative treatments and procedures;
8. Full disclosure of any financial or other type of benefit or incentive received from the manufacturer of any product prescribed as part a treatment plan or any device used for a procedure;
9. Full disclosure of any drug or medical device whereby the FDA approval for marketing was based on clinical research funded and/or controlled by the manufacturer;
10. Full disclosure of all of the manufacturer's warnings, especially when the label states that safety during

pregnancy, for nursing mothers, or use in children under certain ages has not been established.

Additionally, the revised version of PPACA must require health care practitioners who propose treatment plans to take responsibility for making certain that the patient or responsible party understands how to self-administer the treatment plan. The patient teaching must include complete nutritional assessment and guidance as well as other necessary life-style changes such has increasing or curtailing physical activity in a program of regular exercise. Specific instructions must be in printed format in the language that the patient or family member understands. If the at-home treatment plan requires skilled intervention, the physician must refer the patient to a home care case manager to coordinate the services and delivery of required health care products.

Finally, the new revised law must require that the physician make an accurate assessment of the patient's ability to understand how to carry out the prescribed medical regimen and his/her financial ability to acquire all of the necessary supplies, medication and/or equipment. The law should also require that the health care provider make at least one follow-up phone call after the visit to find out if the patient is able to follow the prescribed regimen. Moreover, if any patient or responsible party calls with a question, the medical care providers must be required to reply on the same day of the call.

In summary, legislating basic standards to improve communication will substantially reduce the millions of medical mistakes that occur because the patient was not able to understand the doctors' instructions while the doctor was oblivious to the miscommunication.

Improve the health of the population.

Improving the overall population health is so broad in scope that it must be narrowed down to how reforms in health care provision can accomplish this task. We would also have to include environmental issues, unemployment, immigration, crime, consumer product safety, food supply integrity, quality of potable water, sewage, sanitation, etc.

Accordingly, we shall focus on how improvements in reducing health care disparity between socioeconomic groups will improve population health. The main problem is the disparity in physician fee schedules. Medicare sets the standard for physician compensation, which is about 300 percent more than Medicaid. Therefore, personal prejudices notwithstanding, most doctors in private practice won't accept Medicaid recipients as patients. Consequently, the quality of care is inferior because Medicaid beneficiaries must seek their health care in government owned clinics or outpatient centers run by teaching hospitals that are overburdened with colossal patient loads. The undesirable effects that lower the quality of care in Medicaid clinics are as follows:

1. Waiting more than one month to diagnose new medical problems;
2. Poor communication with little or no follow-up;
3. Lack of continuity because of physician rotations;
4. Higher risk of medical mistakes by inexperienced physicians-in-training;
5. Less time for adequate patient teaching.

The result of such practices is much shorter average life expectancy and an infant mortality rate three times higher than the population that has health coverage through private insurance.

Therefore, the new revised version of PPACA must address the abuses of Government paid health care by doing away with the disparity of the physician fee schedule. What justification can there be for arbitrarily setting Medicaid reimbursement at twenty dollars per visit when Medicare pays sixty dollars? It is pure discrimination against the poor, most of whom are blacks, Hispanics and other minorities. Hence it is unconstitutional as well as immoral and the new health care reform law must do away with such inequity. Once this physician fee disproportion disappears, millions of Medicaid recipients will have access to private physicians and population health will improve.

Additionally preventive care measures are essentially for improving population health. The PPACA has provision for preventive health services that qualifying private insurance companies must provide free of any copays or deductibles such as:

- o Blood pressure, diabetes and cholesterol screening;
- o Many cancer screenings, including mammograms and colonoscopies;
- o Counseling on such topics as quitting smoking, losing weight, eating healthfully;
- o Treating depression; alcoholism and drug addiction;
- o Routine vaccinations against diseases such as measles, polio or meningitis;
- o Flu and pneumonia vaccines;
- o Prenatal care and counseling;
- o Regular well-baby and well-child visits, from birth to age 18.

However, once again we have a large segment of the population deprived of such services because of the disparity between private insurance and Medicaid. Facilities that serve the Medicaid populations are so overburdened with too many patients that they have little time for counseling. Educational campaigns to encourage weight loss, good prenatal care and improved coping with stress and depression among the poor inner city populations are virtually non-existent. The government must impose the same law on itself; otherwise, the new rules governing private insurance are discriminatory and unconstitutional.

Improving the safety and reliability of the U.S. health care system

Over the last ten years, Hospital care alone has caused at least 2,000,000 deaths and three times that many survivable injuries. In order to alleviate this problem and reach the proposed national goal of a safer and more reliable health care system Congress needs to add a new section entitled "Patient Safety Standards" because PPACA is thus far silent on the issue of patient safety. For starters, they can focus on the twenty-eight never-events that Medicare, Medicaid and private insurance companies will refuse to pay for because these are common hospital mistakes that should never happen. We shall focus on those for which standards for prevention can be logistically legislated. There are also other aspects of health care such as institutional mismanagement that need legislative action such as corporate officers being held personally accountable for death and injury due to fiscal recklessness, maintaining dangerous staffing levels and leaving life support equipment in disrepair.

Legislating Patient Safety Standards in Hospitals

The new amendment to PPACA to mandate patient safety standards must require such standards of care that would render those common sentinel events that cause death or serious disability as unlikely to ever occur.

1. Surgery performed on the wrong body part

The standards for prevention should include a preoperative visit during which the surgeon draws the incision line on the skin with a non-toxic marker pen where the surgery is to take place. Additionally, there needs to be a barcode system in use that the nurse can use to verify the planned procedure and body part to ensure that there is no confusion between right and left. There also needs to be a requirement to ask the patient to state his or her understanding of what surgical procedure is to be performed and on which part of the body. The failure to implement these safeguards should result in being liable for criminal negligence.

2. Surgery performed on the wrong patient

Patient identification is simple and straight forward. The patient wears an identification bracelet with a barcode that the circulating nurse can use to match the patient with the chart and the operating room schedule. The patient safety standard amendment must emphasize that failure to properly identify a patient prior to surgery will not be tolerated.

3. Wrong surgical procedure performed on a patient

It would be catastrophic if a person goes in for a gallbladder removal and wakes up missing a healthy kidney and then has to go again to remove the diseased gall bladder. Unfortunately, such a scenario is not so rare. Similar safeguards need to be in place as for the two sentinel events described above with criminal penalties for wanton non-compliance.

4. Unintended retention of a foreign object in a patient after surgery or other procedure

The retention of a foreign object like a sponge, instrument or needle is pure recklessness. The purpose of including this in health care reform legislation is to impress upon the surgeons and nurses the need to remain diligent in counting the items before during and after surgery to make certain that what went into the body cavity was removed before closure. If the count is wrong, there must be an x-ray taken in the O.R. without exception, preferably before final closure. The failure to carry out those simple precautions is reckless endangerment and should carry penalties for criminal negligence.

5. Death or brain damage due to lack of oxygen during anesthesia

The primary responsibility the anesthesiologist or nurse anesthetist is to maintain the patient's airway and provide adequate oxygen. This is especially crucial because during induction the anesthetist administers a drug that paralyzes every muscle in the body rendering the patient incapable of breathing. Therefore, he or she has total control over the patient's respirations. The failure to properly intubate the patient to establish an airway is lethal. Two or three minutes of depriving the brain of oxygen will invariably produce irreversible brain damage. Thus in the interest of public safety the patient safety amendment must contain a mandate to auscultate[44] the lungs

---

[44] Listen with a stethoscope

immediately after intubation. Listening for the movement of air assures that the lungs are being properly aerated. Additionally, there has to be a mandate for make certain that the oxygen line is connected. Finally, there is need for periodic arterial blood gas levels during the course of surgery. If a wanton breach of these basic standards results in death or permanent brain damage, there should be liability for criminal negligence.

6. Death of a basically healthy patient during or within 24 hours of surgery

With the unexpected death or serious disability within 24 hours of surgery of a patient classified as otherwise healthy, one has to suspect that there was an untoward preventable event. The patient safety amendment (PSA) would have to require reporting the death to state and local authorities and conducting investigation as to the cause of death. The results of the investigation must be fully disclosed to the family along with any incident reports or internal memos. Any attempt at cover-up should result in criminal liability.

7. Patient death or serious disability associated with the use of contaminated drugs, devices, or biologics provided by the health care facility

All liquids that patients receive intravenously, into the abdominal cavity or into the spinal canal must be sterile. If there is any contamination prior to infusion, overwhelming infections will occur that can cause death or catastrophic survivable injury. Since contamination occurs because of carelessness, patient safety standards would require strict adherence to the following rules:

1. There must be continuing education programs on sterile technique.
2. Hospitals and other inpatient health care facilities must adhere to manufacturers' storage instructions for maintaining integrity of containers and packages with sterile contents.
3. There must also be infection control of sterile supply storage areas in maintaining a clean environment.
4. Central supply departments must adhere to strict guidelines in the process of re-sterilizing reusable surgical instruments and devices.
5. Sterilizing items for re-use that are intended to be disposable must be strictly prohibited and violators should be held criminally liable.
6. Mixing of intravenous fluids for hyper-alimentation[45] outside of a laminar air-flow device[46] must be strictly prohibited with criminal penalties for non-compliance.

7. Patient death or injury caused by the misuse of a medical device

There are several states that have provisions in their health codes that prohibit using a medical device for some purpose other than for what it is intended. Those codes invariably define medical devices as including but not limited to catheters, drains, and other specialized tubes, infusion pumps, and ventilators. Therefore, the new PSA must include absolute prohibition against using any medical device in any way other than for which it was designed. Non-compliance would have to

---

[45] Intravenous infusion of complete nutrition through a central line
[46] A device that literally sucks the microbes out of the air in an enclosed environment, which can be an entire room or table-top workspace

be considered as a wanton disregard of the patient's safety and well-being.

8. Patient death or serious disability caused by intravascular air embolism occurring in a health care facility

Every time a nurse sets up an intravenous (IV) infusion the tubing that connects the IV solution bag to the vein is filled with air. The nurse must flush the tubing with the solution to remove all of the air before connecting it to the patient's vein access catheter. Once the nurse completes the initial hook-up, there is a continuous problem of air pockets being trapped in the tubing as the solution flows. There is also a frequent problem of air getting into the line after the solution runs out. When that happens, the nurse must remove the air before restarting the infusion with the new bag. A large bolus of air in the veins causes death because when it reaches the lungs it ironically blocks the exchange of oxygen because this air on the wrong side of the fence, so to speak. Small amounts of air like a few tiny bubbles don't cause immediate problems but there is a cumulative effect when air pockets repetitively infuse into the blood stream negligence.

Therefore, the root cause of this complication is a wanton disregard of the patient's safety and well-being. Hence the PSA should establish zero tolerance under federal law for air embolism causing disability or death.

9. Infant discharged to the wrong person

Baby switching accidents happen in hospitals despite the fact that there are enough safeguards with barcoded identification bracelets and foot prints to match the baby with the mom before discharge. That's why the general consensus is that two mothers should never have to go home with the other one's baby. Therefore the PSA must contain the necessary standards as a mandate and hold health care workers personally accountable for willful non-compliance.

10. Patient death or serious disability associated with patient elopement

Hospital and nursing facility patients who are mentally incompetent and not physically disabled are always at risk of wandering off the premises, leading to being run over, dying of exposure or injured in a criminal attack. Most of these people walk out in hospital gowns that are open at the back, so it should be easy to catch them if the entrances and exits are properly guarded. Wandering alarm technology is cheap enough to acquire and should be mandated by law. Hence the failure to provide adequate safeguards is inexcusable and the PSA should reflect that.

11. Patient suicide, or attempted suicide resulting in serious disability in a health care facility

Suicidal behavior is observable and preventable in most cases. The initial nursing assessment upon admission must invariably contain a behavioral component that screens for depression and expression of suicidal ideas. However, since a new onset of suicidal behavior can't always be anticipated, the PSA should mandate a thorough investigation to determine if the nurse performed the required behavioral assessment and took all reasonable precaution measures that were available to identify suicidal tendencies and implement preventive measures. There also needs to be a requirement to fully disclose the results of the investigation to the patient's family or responsible person including incident reports and internal memos. Cover-up attempts must result in criminal liability.

Additionally, every patient unit must be designed to prevent unexpected attempts at suicide such as privacy curtains that will fall to the floor with any weight attached over a few pounds, and shatter proof windows that cannot be opened more than a few inches. The rooms also have to be free of glass objects, flammable liquids such as rubbing alcohol and matches or lighters. There must also be screening for any personal items that can be used to self-inflict wounds like knives, razors and guns.

12. Patient death or serious disability associated with a medication error

Medical errors involve the wrong drug, wrong dose, wrong patient, wrong time, wrong rate, wrong preparation, or wrong route of administration. Such errors can be eliminated with the appropriate technology. The correct standard is for hospital pharmacies to send unit doses of prescribed medication to the nurses with the patient's barcoded identification on the drug pack or container. The nurses match the drug barcode with the id bracelet and voila—the right patient every time with the correct drug dosage according to the doctor's orders, which are in the computer system. Such systems must be mandated for every hospital and nursing facility. However, the right route of administration is still up to the nurse, so the PSA must prohibit administering a particular medication through any means other than what the manufacturer intended.

13. Patient death or serious disability caused by mismatching blood types for transfusions

All blood transfusions are potentially lethal. The patient's blood type has to be an exact match to the blood or byproduct or the patient suffers a hemolytic reaction which is incompatible with life. Those who survive after a complete blood exchange suffer serious damage to vital organs. Such sentinel events are indeed tragic because there is no legitimate reason for them. The standard that should be incorporated into the PSA is for two registered nurses to check the serial number and blood type between the blood product and the patient's identification bracelet which contains the same information. It's a simple failsafe, so when the nurses fail to comply it should qualify as criminal negligence. If the blood was mislabeled then there must be an investigation to find out where the breakdown occurred.

14. Maternal death or serious disability associated with labor or delivery in a low-risk pregnancy

Low risk pregnancy with unexpected maternal complications is a clear indication that the mother either had a potential problem that was not diagnosed or attended to during gestation or that there was a screw-up during labor and delivery that caused an adverse event or reaction. The key purpose of legislation area is prevention. Complications can arise at any time during labor and the result can be anything from a baby and mother to maternal and fetal death depending on how fast and efficiently the medical and nursing staff responds.

Thus, certain safety standards have to be instituted like minimum nurse staffing and a requirement for the obstetrician to be on premises at all times during labor. The common practice of leaving the hospital with instructions to the nurse to "Call me when the contractions are five minutes apart;" just doesn't cut it. Moreover, the fetal monitors have to be in good working order and if there are any abnormalities, the nurse must notify the doctor immediately. When there are nurse-midwives on staff, there must be a supervising obstetrician on call for any complications. Since there still continues to be a death rate among low-risk mothers at child birth, such safety standards must be part of the PSA.

15. Patient death or serious disability associated with hypoglycemia, occurring in a health care facility

Hypoglycemic shock (dangerously low blood sugar) only occurs when someone with insulin-dependent diabetes receives an overdose of insulin or fails to eat sufficient amounts of carbohydrates to maintain the blood sugar at safe levels. When a low-blood sugar crisis occurs, this is the result of a failure on the part of the nurses to balance the food intake with the administration of insulin. Thus, the patient safety standards must include blood glucose monitoring before administering insulin and anticipation of food needs that will counterbalance the peak effect with long-acting insulin. Individuals who cause death and injury by wanton failure to comply must be held accountable.

16. Death or serious disability associated with

failure to identify and treat elevated bilirubin in neonates (kernicterus)

Elevated bilirubin is a common affliction among newborns. They appear jaundice in the first days of life and require phototherapy. All babies must be screened for bilirubin levels during the first day of life. The fact that many babies are still dying because of a failure to perform a simple routine blood test or the failure to apply phototherapy for a few days is intolerable. Why Obama and company would refuse to eliminate this criminal negligence baby-killing as part of the new national priority is incomprehensible. Therefore the PSA must include a mandate of personal criminal liability for anyone who fails to comply with screening all neonates for elevated bilirubin and treating those who need it.

17. Pressure ulcers acquired after admission to a health care facility

Pressure ulcers are a huge problem in health care that affects about 10 percent of all those admitted to hospitals and 25 percent in nursing facilities. At present, Medicaid and Medicare reimbursement policies require that pressure ulcers develop to stage III, which is exposure of muscle, before they will pay for a special mattress that is designed to prevent pressure ulcers. Thus government is contributing significantly to the problem. Therefore the PSA must put an end to such policies that cause injury and death as well as increasing the cost of care.

Additionally, there two basic standards of care that need legislative attention such as turning the patient every two hours and keeping the skin clean and dry. The common place stories of people dying with multiple bedsores with infection and gangrene down to the bone are intolerable, yet they keep happening. There are some who defend themselves by saying that bedsores can't be prevented; if so, then let them show that they provided the basic care required for prevention by documenting that they turned their patients every two hours without fail and that those patients who were incontinent were kept clean and dry at all times.

18. Patient death or serious disability due to spinal manipulative therapy

Spinal manipulation requires skill acquired by training. Only chiropractors and doctors of osteopathy are qualified to perform such maneuvers. When properly done with the necessary skill, injury should not occur. Therefore, no one should be allowed to perform such a procedure without the proper credentials. An unqualified person who performs such manipulation causing paralysis or death must face criminal liability.

19. Patient death or serious disability associated with an electric shock or electrical cardioversion in a health care facility

There are two standards that will prevent most deaths related to correcting lethal heart rhythms with electric shock. The first is that the type of electric shock delivery must be appropriate to the diagnosis. The second is that the equipment must be in good repair. For example, defibrillation is only appropriate for ventricular fibrillation. If the doctor misapplies it the patient will go into cardiac arrest. If the machine does not deliver the right amount of electricity (measures in Joules) the patient will likely die. There are no exceptions and no room for error. Additionally, cardioversion is even trickier because the shock has to be delivered at a certain point during the heartbeat. For this the doctor must rely on the equipment to work properly. The PSA amendment must require that equipment be in good repair at all times.

20. Any incident in which an oxygen line (or other type of gas) contains the wrong gas or is contaminated by toxic substances

It's difficult to believe that such mishaps would occur on a regular basis. There must be basic engineering protocols that establish that only qualified technicians would have access to the source of gases administered in a health care facility. There must also be mandates for frequent safety inspections both at the source and at all of the points of delivery. Patient rooms should not have any gas other than oxygen. Other types of gases are only administered by anesthesiologists or nurse anesthetists. The multiline devices that they use must be checked for safety before each use to make certain that the different gas lines are correctly color coded and labeled.

21. Patient death or serious disability associated with a burn incurred from any source while being cared for in a health care facility

Scalding beverages and hot soaks cause most thermal injuries hospitals and nursing homes. Sometimes flash fires occur from lighting a match or cigarette lighter in a room with a high concentration of oxygen. The preventive safety protocols are simple; measure the temperature of all heated liquids and do not bring it to the patient if the temperature is more than 110 degrees

Fahrenheit. However, such accidents occur with astounding regularity because there is no accountability for such wanton carelessness.

22. Patient death or serious disability associated with a fall in a health care facility

Patients fall every day in virtually every hospital and nursing facility. The current standards of care require that every patient receive a fall risk assessment and that interventions for prevention be in place depending on the level of risk. The health care managers resign themselves to believing that not all falls are preventable and they have a legal defense when they can show that the patient fell despite the exercise of reasonable precautions. Once health care management develops a zero tolerance for falls, then all falls can become preventable. The only way to prevent almost all falls is to have one person sitting with each patient at all times. A staff of volunteers could be utilized to perform sitter services. There is no shortage of volunteers in most areas as all high school students need a certain number of community service hours to graduate and there plenty of people given the opportunity for community service in lieu of jail time for minor offenses. Therefore, the PSA should mandate that volunteers be assigned to every patient unit to perform safety precaution services to prevent falling.

23. Patient death or serious disability associated with the use of restraints or bedrails in a health care facility

Because of the number of people who were hanged or lost their limbs because of improper use of standard restraints or the use of makeshift materials to tie people down, those states that have adopted the uniform public health code have added rules and regulations in the use of restraints. Moreover, bedrails also cause problems because people try to climb over or slip around them. When patient falls with the bedrail involved it usually exacerbates the trauma. The rules regarding restraints and bedrails are clear and every nurse knows that when he/she violates those rules death or disability ensues. Therefore, willful non-compliance cannot be tolerated any longer.

24. Any health care service provided by or on the orders of a non-licensed individual

No patient or family member should expect to be the victim of a quack. However, despite that we have laws that are supposed to protect us from such criminal activity, it still happens. It's one thing for people in a community to find out that a "doctor" was practicing without a license after some time, but to be in a hospital and find that a quack has been prescribing medicine or preforming invasive procedures is frightening. The new PSA must address this issue and require that safety precautions be followed with zero tolerance for willful non-compliance. Every health care provider should be required to show their credentials on demand to the patient or family member. Hospitals should be required to provide their patients with pamphlets with instructions on how to access the state licensing agency website to check to see if any individual's license is valid. Finally, every staff person who encounters an unfamiliar provider must take the name of the stranger and verify his/her authorization to be in that location providing services.

25. Abduction of a patient of any age

Hospitals and nursing facilities are responsible for the safety of their patients or residents; this includes preventing abduction. Such crimes can be avoided by requiring that every patient being discharged be accompanied by a staff member to the exit. If the patient refuses to comply, then security personnel at all exist must be notified to make an assessment as to whether the patient is leaving of his or her own accord. The PSA must require that all health care facilities orient their staff to guard against abduction and know where their patients are at all times. When patients have to be moved to other parts of the hospital for tests or procedures, there must be a system of verifying that the patient has safely reached the intended destination.

26. Sexual assault on a patient within or on the grounds of the health care facility

Sexual assault on a patient in a health care facility is especially tragic because when people enter into these environments there is an expectation of being able to trust the staff. People often find themselves with their modesty compromised when examined and treated by medical personnel. Health care management personnel have an absolute obligation to provide criminal background screening on all hires and contractors who have access to patient areas. There also must be adequate security precautions of taking down the identification of every visitor. The practice of printing temporary picture identification for every visitor as done in some hospitals must be standardized by Federal law. There are too many facilities in which the security is shabby or non-existent. It is not enough to hold criminally negligent managers liable, these types of attacks must be prevented.

27. Physical assault of a patient in a health care facility resulting in death or significant injury

All too often staff members who have total power and control over patients commit physical and verbal abuse and then try to use intimidation to make their victims keep silent. The elderly in nursing homes and psychiatric patients are especially vulnerable, although such crimes occur in general hospitals as well. Careful screening of employees and contractors can prevent almost all occurrences with the kind of technology that exists today in law enforcement communities. Facilities that have a history of patient abuse should be required to give full disclosure to the public of the number of incidences and on which units in the manner that restaurants face public disclosure of non-compliance with health codes that put customers at risk. The PSA should also give the government the authority to put any health care facility into receivership to replace the governing body and management personnel for non-compliance with patient safety laws. Public safety must be the first priority as it is with the airline and food service industries.

Care Coordination

The fourth newly recommended national priority is to ensure that patients receive well-coordinated care within and across all health care organizations, settings, and levels of care. The new age of medical specialization has made it particularly hazardous to patients because different specialists are prescribing medications often not knowing what other doctors will prescribe. There is most often no communication between different specialists because the primary care physician (PCP) refers the patient and does the communicating. Thus, the heart specialist and the foot doctor will most probably never speak to each other because they will not see any reason for a provider team conference. However, each one has the authority to prescribe medications without knowing what the other doctors intend to prescribe. Consequently, there are untold thousands of people each year who suffer death or debilitating injury from drug interactions or debilitating central nervous system depression from multiple drugs called "polypharmacy."

Palliative Care

The fifth proposed new national priority is for the amended PPACA to "guarantee appropriate and compassionate care for patients with life-limiting illnesses." To be cautious, one should be aware that there is a lot of political correctness packed into the quoted statement. This quote from the IOM is referring to hospice care, which as it is presented currently, is a means of stopping all manner of expensive treatment in exchange for receiving large doses of Morphine and waiting for death. In such situations it is impossible to rule out assisted suicide or euthanasia since lethal amounts of pain killers are conveniently available in the privacy of the patient's home. Medical examiners do not get involved when a person with terminal illness dies a few months before the doctors' expectations unless there is obvious evidence of a homicide, like a smoking gun with a confession.

Therefore, although end of life care is an important part of the system, it should always be a matter of choice and the decision should never be irreversible or require that the patient lose all hope of survival. In fact I have been working with a hospice organization that does not stand in the way of continuing treatment or bringing in complimentary alternative medicine

(CAM). We have established this program in my community and we call it "hospice with hope." The idea hit me when I was sitting with my friend and client, Sam (of blessed memory) at his oncologist's office. He had advanced cancer in his pancreas, liver and lungs. The doctor said, "The chemo therapy didn't work. There is nothing more that can be done, so I am recommending that you go into hospice care."

Sam stared at the doctor with a stone like expression on his face in response to this shocking news and replied, "That's a death sentence."

I interjected with, "Doctor, are you saying nothing can be done, or that there is nothing that you know of that will help."

The doctor replied, "There is nothing that I personally know of to treat this condition."

At that point, Sam decided to enter into the world of alternative medicine, but it was too late because the chemotherapy had wrecked his appetite and nutritional status and caused him to suffer from dehydration and starvation syndrome; which, of course, destroyed his natural ability to fight the cancer with the help of herbs, and other recognized methodologies. In retrospect, there should have at least been a concerted effort to protect Sam's nutritional status during the chemotherapy with herbal and nutritional supplements. Without these considerations the entire concept of "palliative" care becomes nothing more than a tool for a death panel.

Eliminating Overuse

The sixth of the new national health care reform priorities is eliminating overuse. More precisely, overuse refers to duplication of services and higher than necessary level of care, such as hospitalizing people who can be treated in a sub-acute nursing facility or as outpatients. The former is straight forward and the PPACA Patient Safety Amendment (PSA) can easily contain wording that would prohibit doctors from ordering unnecessary diagnostic tests such as lab work, X-rays and scans. As mentioned previously, let's say a primary care physician has obtained blood work and X-rays and then referred the patient to a specialist because some of the results were abnormal. If the specialist orders a repeat of the tests as a matter of policy for all newly referred patients that is a duplication of services. The PSA can easily abolish this practice by making the doctors pay for any such duplicate diagnostic testing.

The second component of overuse is providing more expensive higher levels of care than what the patient needs. For example, intensive care versus regular hospital floor is a serious problem regarding overuse. However, there is the question of patient safety vis-à-vis staffing issues. A physician is going to be reluctant to transferring a patient to a regular floor from the ICU knowing that the floor units are understaffed to the point of being dangerous. On the other hand, one area of overuse that is more easily discernible, as mentioned previously, is the practice of transferring nursing home residents to hospitals for minor health problems that can be treated safely at the nursing home. This practice must be abolished by directing the CMS to change its reimbursement policies.

Universal Health Care Access

The seventh new national health care priority is to ensure that all segments of the U.S. population have equal access. When Obama went along with eliminating the public option as a compromise to stop the insurance lobby from turning the legislative effort into the unavoidable train wreck that it became, he destroyed the hope of universal access. Undeniably, we have the some of the best medical technology in the world, but about half the population does not have access to all of it. For the bottom third of this multi-tier system, health care is no better than most third world countries who have no coverage for 95 percent of their population other than poorly equipped government hospitals. Thus there are millions in the United States who are dying or becoming disabled from treatable conditions.

Therefore the big political debate is over the question of "What is the moral imperative of our society?" Is it okay to deny access to 50 million people because they are either self-employed, underemployed, unemployed or depend on Medicaid, or can we find some common ground where the bottom rungs can get more while those at the top make do with a little less? The answer depends on who you ask. The leftists have no problem with causing a train wreck because they don't like the fact that some cars are restricted to those who can pay for first class and the conservatives want no part of any equalization effort that might derail the first class compartments. However, since the health care system in its current state will destroy our economy in the next two decades even with the inequalities unresolved, we have to focus on making it more cost effective before we can equalize all disparities.

Centralize Health Informatics

Although centralized patient health data has its advantages, it puts our privacy in peril. Our health information is supposed to be private and not accessible to anyone other than those whom we authorize. When our charts are digitized and stored in the doctor's computer system, they will be sent over the internet to a central government-owned main-frame. Then we will lose all expectation of privacy because members of the government's law enforcement and intelligence community will have access in the interest of national security. One would have to ask, "What do grandma's gall stones have to do with national security?" However, private information is the best way to gain command and control over people's lives and the specifics don't matter.

On the other hand, our privacy is pretty much a thing of the past for anyone who uses the internet. How many times have we had to clean out adware from our hard drives? Those are the little bugs that keep track of our favorite sites and purchases. How many of those little buggers are on everybody's personal computer that our virus software can't detect? Chances are that the government already has a complete profile on everything about everybody who owns a computer such as bank accounts, investments, real property, purchases, favorite books, favorite movies and all kinds of personal habits. What if they find out about somebody's hemorrhoids? Will they tag that poor soul as a terrorist? Thus there doesn't seem to be much of a risk anymore regarding privacy issues because privacy is a thing of the past and the prevention of medical errors with physician access to a new patient's complete medical history will save a lot of lives.

Wrap Up

Ironically, a group of small voices within the massive bureaucracy in the Obama administration actually came up with a workable solution to the health care debacle. The original whistle blower, Dr. Harvey V. Fineberg, president of the Institute of Medicine actually stayed on and introduced an eight point plan called the "New National Priorities". Astoundingly it could actually work if Obama or anyone in Congress paid attention to it. The plan calls for legislative action to improve patient involvement in the decision making process, engage in preventive action for early detection and treatment, reduce medical and nursing errors, eliminate duplication of services, create hospice with hope, eliminate unnecessary procedures, provide universal access and employ digital health care informatics.

Unfortunately, the proposed eight national priorities in Dr. Finberg's Future National Directions Committee report is nothing more than a footnote. It's a matter of public record and it is sitting in the archives of the Department of Health and Human Services, hidden in plain sight. However, we, the public can change that by emailing copies of the eight national priorities to every member of Congress with a note saying that this is how we can achieve real health care reform. Obama challenged us to recommend ways to improve PPACA apparently without even knowing about the report that came from his own government experts, like Dr. Fineberg. Are you in or out?

17. The Baby-Boomers' Survival Guide

We have to learn what to do in case of the "unlikely" event that government does not follow the common sense approach to health care reform. Picture in the not too distant future that the federal government must make a desperate move to save the economy from total collapse by eliminating the largest single expenditure—institutional health care for those with diminished mental capacity, advanced age over 75 or end stage disease. Logistically, the act of shutting down life support is going to be relatively easy because the largest payer of hospital and nursing facility care is the Medicare system and the chief policy maker is the director of the Centers for Medicare and Medicaid Services (CMS) who serves at the pleasure of the president of the United States.

To continue, there is no question that if health care reform does not take an entirely different course in the next five years, most of us will not have access to any artificial life support care with feeding tubes and ventilators. The new reality will thrust us all into the past; to a time during which such technology was non-existent. The only difference is that we can now use the internet to learn how to deal with the absence of institutional care.

The Rationing of Ventilators and Stomach Tubes

In many instances we will not be able to save our loved ones. Those who remain on institutional life support when the policy changes take effect will perish. The government will simply issue orders to pull the machine plugs and yank out stomach tubes. The Florida courts already established the legal precedent in the Terry Schialvo case by ordering the doctors to remove her feeding tube and let her starve to death. In the health care world of life or death, cash is king. Money drives the life support machines and the personnel to run them. The number of people on life support or who are in an extended coma or "vegetative state" is unknown. The National Center for Health Statistics (NCHS), a branch of the Centers for Disease Control and Prevention (CDC) reported in 2003 that 146,000 permanent feeding tubes were being inserted into people[47]. According to the Brain Injury Association there are approximately 40,000 people diagnosed with being in a persistent vegetative state [48]. Therefore when the Secretary of Health and Human Services decides that it is time to "pull the plug" on mentally non-viable institutionalized patients and those with less than a certain life expectancy, millions of people will die in a single day. Following that some 200,000 people each year will be on the "who shall die" list because the government will declare that life support for people with terminal or long term debilitating illness is improper.

The procedure for placing a stomach tube takes about 20 minutes and requires the use of a hospital operating room. The cost per person is about $12,000 and at the rate of 146,000 per year the total cost is approximately 1.752 billion dollars per year. Since the reason for placing such a tube is the inability to swallow, the stomach tube makes the difference between staying alive or starving to death. Under the new health care reform law the Secretary of Health and Human Services will have discretion

---

[47]   ttp:// hwww.cdc.gov/nchs/dhcs.htm
[48]   http://www.biausa.org/

to decide who can get one and who can't for about 146,000 people per year. This is different from the Schialvo case in which the court determined that there was sufficient evidence to determine that Schialvo had expressed her preference for starving to death rather than remain in a permanent "vegetative" state.

Moreover, the medical community has already capitulated to the idea of denying insertion of stomach tubes to those with less than a certain life expectancy. Regarding the criteria for approving such a procedure, the American College of Gastroenterology had this to say: "A percutaneous endoscopic gastrostomy (PEG) is a procedure for placing a feeding tube directly into the stomach through a small incision in the abdominal wall using an instrument known as an endoscope. The procedure is performed as a means of providing nutrition to patients who cannot take food by mouth. . .When a patient is being considered for PEG tube placement, the patient's life expectancy after the tube is placed needs to be considered to determine if placement of a feeding tube is appropriate. . ."[49]

Thus, this physician group's statement begs the question, "Who will determine what the life expectancy should be in order to consider the procedure as being appropriate?" This also begs the question, "What is a life worth?" The answer is that it depends on who's it is. Aside from the issues of living wills, the new health care mandates will remove the right to choose because spending trillions of dollars per year to keep people alive past a certain age, to perpetuate a "vegetative state" or to maintain life during the "end stage" of a terminal illness will no

---

49 http://www.acg.gi.org/patients/gihealth/peg.asp

longer be an option.

Therefore, for the chronically ill, the inability to swallow will mark the beginning of the end. The insertion of a stomach tube will no longer be an option to prolong life because in the new reality the healthcare providers will have to justify the cost with life-expectancy and a productivity index beyond an arbitrary threshold. However, there will be at least half a million people with stomach tubes at the time that the government implements its plan of systematically removing them. Those who have no family support system are at the mercy of their federally funded caretakers who will have no choice but to follow the dictates of their purse-strings. Those who have a support system will be able to survive with the requisite amount of time and money; time to provide the care and money to buy the supplies and equipment. But because of the ever-present danger of overfilling the stomach, there is a continuous risk of choking during the feedings. However, one can avoid the aspiration of stomach contents by taking a few simple precautions:

1. Always keep the patient's head elevated at 30 degrees during feedings;
2. Check the amount of residual stomach volume by attaching a 50 cc syringe to the stomach tube and drawing back on the plunger to remove and measure the amount of fluid in the stomach;
3. Keep a suction machine with a tonsilar tip at the bedside at all times;
4. In case of vomiting, turn the patient on one side and keep the mouth and throat clear of liquid using the suction machine.

Staying Alive

So, here we are, as I find myself, age 63, a baby boomer along with about one third of the U.S. population knowing that there probably won't be any hospital care available for those of us who are lucky enough to reach age 75 unless there is real healthcare reform. In either event who needs it anyway? As of now if a person is over 60 years of age and needs to go in the hospital now there is a 40% chance that he or she will suffer disabling injury or death from medical or nursing mistakes; so who needs it anyway? Therefore, we have to gear up for staying away from hospitals by preventing those accidents and illness that bring us there. Consequently, what we do now will have its impact in ten years and will determine whether we live or die.

The way to stay healthy and thriving through the golden years requires a support system, focusing on the body, the mind and spirit with family, mind-body preventive maintenance and environmental safety

Family

First, a support system means family. We have to re-establish the family unit as the foundation of our society. Older folks don't normally live in family units in our present culture. They become outcast and end up in nursing homes at the mercy of shady profiteers and government regulators. The development of group home assisted living houses over the last three decades lays a good foundation for developing family units, but we need real caring advocates who will pay attention to our needs. Most of the time our adult children become the advocates. It doesn't mean that children have to become their parents' caretakers, but to live into the future that we are facing, we need to set social actions in motion that will change the inevitable bleak outcome. Therefore, those with parents of advanced age need to form focus groups to meet and discuss ways and means to protect the health and maintain the quality of life of their loved ones.

Mind-Body Maintenance and Disease Prevention

The subject of disease prevention could fill several books, but in the context of baby boomers surviving without hospitals, we need to cover the essentials of good eating and stress reduction. In this perspective, we have to focus on the immune system. That's basically the blood, but several of the vital organs like the skin, liver, spleen and kidneys play a role. There are a lot of buzz words out in cyberspace like free radicals and antioxidants. As we explore these words we will develop some understanding of how we can avoid the preventable common diseases that plague us as we get older.

First, with regard to the anti-aging buzz words like "antioxidants" and "free radicals," the free radical theory of aging implies that antioxidants such as Vitamins A, C, and E, and superoxide dismutase will slow the process of aging by preventing free radicals from oxidizing sensitive biological molecules or reducing the formation of free radicals. The antioxidant chemicals found in many foods are frequently cited as the basis of claims for the benefits of a high intake of vegetables and fruits in the diet. However, we really don't have any hard evidence that eating blueberries, strawberries and other fruits and vegetables is going to extend our life-spans. Nonetheless, a complete vitamin intake through healthy foods and supplements is vital to staying out of hospitals. In any event, we need to focus more on disease prevention than extending life expectancy. Although these are mutually inclusive concepts, with the former we need to understand that the most common preventable diseases that cause hospital dependence in people over 65 years of age are heart disease, pneumonia, uncontrolled diabetes and injuries from falling. Therefore, we shall now discuss those in terms of prevention.

Heart Matters

Heart attack is the number one natural killer across the board for the most part not because the heart wears out at a specific age, but due to blockage of the coronary circulation that provides blood supply to the heart muscles. Most of those blockages develop from dietary misadventures over a life time, causing a slow buildup of plaque (fatty deposits) that either closes off one or more of the coronary vessels or causes blood clots because the plaque acts like fly paper with red blood cells. Therefore we have to be concerned about cholesterol and heart healthy diets consisting of fish oil, oatmeal and vitamin supplements. It is also vital to visit a cardiologist to establish a baseline of heart information and get on a prevention regimen which must include regular exercise.

Additionally biofeedback techniques to measure heart rate and blood pressure during deep breathing and meditation are useful to reduce stress that overtaxes the heart. Learning to lower blood pressure and heart rate at will is an easy process. It's a matter of understanding the parasympathetic nerve response and how to stimulate it. Take a deep breath and let the air out slowly against some resistance that you create by bearing down slightly as you normally do when you move your bowels. This increases pressure within the chest and abdomen and triggers the parasympathetic response which lowers heart rate and blood pressure. You will need a digital blood pressure machine to measure pressure and heart rate while you do this exercise. It will take some practice, but it is easy to accomplish.

Moreover, most standard heart disease prevention literature will tell you that you need a minimum of a thirty minute aerobic workout three times per week to keep your cardiovascular system in good working order. I always shy away from making such general statements because for many that is not nearly enough and for some it may be too much. Exercise programs need to be tailored to the individual. If you are a member of the baby-boomer generation, it's best to begin with a stress test if you haven't had one recently and ask your doctor to recommend a starting point with gradual increases. If you can't or won't consult a doctor, just stay as physically active as you can without over exerting yourself. Be especially careful about engaging in a sudden increase of physical labor such as shoveling your driveway after a snowstorm, which could be a heart attack waiting to happen.

Preventing Pneumonia

The respiratory system is particularly vulnerable to infection in the elderly because physical activity naturally slows down. Moreover, if there is progressive arthritis in the joints causing pain with normal movement, then the person tends to slow down even further becoming progressively more sedentary. This results in shallow breathing and pooling of secretions within the lungs, which in turn creates a haven for viruses and bacteria. The final result is pneumonia. Therefore, the best prevention is to keep moving with deep breathing and coughing exercises several times per day. The key is to keep the secretions moving and expel them periodically.

Being alone and increasingly less mobile is potentially catastrophic. There must at least be some emotional support and encouragement from others. People need to learn how to give each other basic chest therapy by tapping on the upper and lower back with cupped hands to loosen secretions while the receiving person takes deep breaths and coughs. The process must be repeated until the person expectorates some sputum. If one listens to the chest one can hear gurgling sounds if there is some mucous that needs to be expelled in this manner. Paying close attention to a person's activity and respiratory status in this manner will go a long way to prevent pneumonia.

Controlling Blood Sugar

The onset of diabetes is largely unavoidable in older folks. Everyone has a finite amount of insulin production which is genetically determined. It's just like fuel in a tank. The more you use, the faster it runs out. Therefore, the less we indulge in bleached flour and sugar, the longer the insulin will last. Thus, those baby-boomers who are not diabetic also need to severely curtail their intake of white bread, candy, cookies, cake, ice cream and the like. It's not as easy as it sounds, but we have to keep thinking of the unintended consequences of sweet-tooth binges. Remember the goal is to live life to the fullest without going into the hospital because we can expect that hospital care will soon be unavailable to people over 75, and even while we still have access, we have to face the fact that hospital mistakes accidentally kill one in every fifty patients with most of the victims being over 65 years of age.

For those who have diabetes, controlling blood sugar requires effort and diligence. Glucose, the simplest form of sugar is the fuel that sustains life at the cellular level. There must a level between 90 and 120 milligrams per deciliter (one tenth of a liter) for any person to stay alive. Glucose is what remains of the cane sugar and other carbohydrates after the digestive system breaks them down. The cells draw the glucose (fuel) from the blood to burn as needed. The body needs insulin to be able to move the glucose from the blood vessels to the cells. Thus, the individual with diabetes has two challenges. The first is to either stimulate more insulin production or take synthetic insulin to utilize the glucose and keep it from accumulating to dangerously high levels in the blood (hyperglycemia). The other challenge is to make certain that there is no overcompensation which would cause the glucose to drop to dangerously low levels (hypoglycemia). The diabetic person has to monitor his/her blood glucose levels with a glucometer. These are readily available at most drug stores and are easy to use. Older folks need to partner up with each other to provide reminders and other assistance as needed. Keeping the blood glucose under control will go a long way to sustaining a healthy life and avoid other complications like blindness and loss of limbs.

Intervention for Fall Prevention

The statistics on injuries from falling in the 65 and over population is alarming, especially when we consider that those terrible numbers are under-reported[50]. About one third of the population over the age of 65 falls each year, and the risk of falls increases until at 80 years and older, over half of the seniors fall annually. Thus we can see that current methods of prevention are a dismal failure. Additionally, the risk of falling increases once an older person has fallen. Fifty-three percent of those who fall are two to three times more likely to fall again.

To continue, falls among the elderly account for 25% of all hospital admissions and 40% of all nursing home admissions. Moreover, 40% of those admitted do not return to independent living and 25% die within a year of the fall. Therefore, fall prevention is the most important intervention to remain free of institutional dependence.

The first step in preventing a commonly occurring event is to assess the risk. Those conditions that most often lead to falling are as follows:
1. confusion;
2. agitation or other aberrant behavior;
3. diabetes;
4. physical impairment, such as with a history of stroke;
5. balance impairment, as with inner ear inflammation;
6. low blood pressure (postural hypotension);
7. history of fainting (syncope);
8. history of epilepsy;
9. visual impairment;
10. frequent urge to urinate;
11. diarrhea;

---

[50] http://www.learnnottofall.com/content/fall-facts/how-often.jsp

12. incontinence;
13. prior falls;
14. taking sedatives, hypnotics, narcotics, and the like;
15. neurological diseases such as Parkinson's and multiple sclerosis.

Unfortunately, even people in excellent health also fall because of human error in the course of normal activity. People with one or more of the above risk factors will inevitably fall unless there is someone to provide constant supervision. There is no way around that. For the past few decades until now we have grown to depend on the federal, state and local governments to take care of our elderly. In other developing countries like the Philippines, the family is the strongest unit of their society. Nursing homes are virtually unheard of because people respect their older family members and take care of them. With the economy on the verge of collapse, our government cannot take care of the senior citizens. That gravy train is soon coming to a grinding halt. Within the next five years we will have to take care of our own parents and grandparents or they die; it's that simple.

Here are a few tips for fall prevention in the home:
1. Keep hallways and stairs well lighted;
2. Bathrooms must have hand rails;
3. Eliminate throw rugs;
4. If there is any incontinence or frequent urination use a bedside commode;
5. Keep floors clear of loose items;
6. Use call devices that the senior person can wear on a necklace or wrist band;
7. Orient the older person at bed time as to the surroundings location of the bathroom;

8. Use motion sensors to alert family members when a senior person is moving outside a predetermined "safe zone."

Wrap UP

At the closing of this book during the summer of 2011, the United States Supreme Court has rejected the application for a fast track decision made by Florida and 24 other states. They ruled that the constitutionality of the Patient Protection and Affordable Care Act (PPACA) of 2010 will have to be decided through the normal appeals process of each level of the federal court system. As such, we will would not know the outcome of this constitutional battle until July of 2012.

However, the fact that PPACA survived the constitutional challenge is academic. We are still stuck with a bloated over-priced health care industry that kills more people than the diseases it treats while being run like a criminal enterprise complete with government corruption. The bottom line is that we still have to push for real health care reform to reduce the carnage by making it safer. Moreover, while a shift in families taking care of their elders rather than pushing them off on the government would be a positive result, we have to stop this insane plan to deny hospital care to the elderly and setting panels to determine who shall live and who shall die.

Thus far, we live in a society that sanctifies life and holds it sacred. We cannot revert leaving our elders to fend for themselves and languish without proper care. If we do that we destroy our humanity and set ourselves up to become euthanized when a panel of cold hearted bureaucrats decides that we no longer have anything worthwhile to contribute to society. It won't matter that we can make a significant difference in the lives of our grandchildren with love, affection, moral guidance and education. We all would become a mere statistic with our lives clicked away by a passionless bean-counter who decides that for those of us who have reached the age of seventy-five, a few more years of living is not worth the investment.

Rather than continue with this inane policy of elder abandonment to reduce health costs, It is time for us to find ways for our senior citizens who have been cast aside to make their invaluable contributions. They can be surrogate grandparents to the countless numbers of children who are likewise outcast and provide loving guidance with the benefit of their wisdom from life experiences. Causing elderly castaways to start feeling needed and useful is by far the best possible anti-aging and preventive medicine program.

www.ingramcontent.com/pod-product-compliance
Lightning Source LLC
Chambersburg PA
CBHW061502180526
45171CB00001B/8